A.S. Fauci · G. Pantaleo (Eds.)

Immunopathogenesis of HIV Infection

Springer
Berlin
Heidelberg
New York
Barcelona
Budapest
Hong Kong
London
Milan
Paris
Santa Clara
Singapore
Tokyo

A.S. Fauci   G. Pantaleo (Eds.)

Immunopathogenesis of HIV Infection

With 18 Figures and 7 Tables

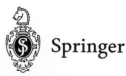 Springer

Anthony S. Fauci
Laboratory of Immunoregulation
National Institute of Allergy and Infectious Diseases
National Institutes of Health
10 Center Drive MSC 1876
Building 10, Room 11B13
Bethesda, MD 20892-1876
USA

Giuseppe Pantaleo
Laboratory of AIDS Immunopathogenesis
Department of Medicine
Division of Infectious Diseases
Centre Hospitalier Universitaire Vadois (CHUV)
1011 Lausanne
Switzerland

ISBN 3-540-63254-9 Springer-Verlag Berlin Heidelberg New York

Library of Congress Cataloging-in-Publication Data applied for

Die Deutsche Bibliothek – CIP-Einheitsaufnahme

Immunopathogenesis of HIV infection : with 7 tables / A. S. Fauci ; G. Pantaleo (ed.). - Ber lin ;
Heidelberg ; New York : Springer, 1997
I-sBN 3-540-63254-9

Production: PRO EDIT GmbH, D-69126 Heidelberg
Typesetting: Satztechnik K. Steingräber, D-69126 Heidelberg
Cover Design: design & production GmbH, D-69121 Heidelberg

SPIN: 10633782   27/3136-5 4 3 2 1 0 - Printed on acid-free paper

Contens

List of Contributors

Bolognesi, D. P.
Departement of Surgery, Box 2926, Duke University Medical Center, Durham, NC 27710, USA

Chen, D.-H.
Departement of Surgery, Box 2926, Duke University Medical Center, Durham, NC 27710, USA

Cohen, O. J.
Laboratory of Immunoregulation, National Institute of Allergy and Infectious Diseases, National Institutes of Health, 10 Center Drive MSC 1876, Building 10, Room 11B13, Bethesda, MD 20892-1876, USA

Fauci, A. S.
Laboratory of Immunoregulation, National Institute of Allergy and Infectious Diseases, National Institutes of Health, 10 Center Drive MSC 1876, Building 10, Room 11B13, Bethesda, MD 20892-1876, USA

Greenberg, M. L.
Departement of Surgery, Box 2926, Duke University Medical Center, Durham, NC 27710, USA

Havlir, D. V.
University of California, San Diego, Departement of Medicine and Pathology and the San Diego Veterans Affairs Medical Center, San Diego, Californa, USA

Jassoy, C.
Institute for Virology and Immunobiology, Julius-Maximilians University, Würzburg, Germany

Koup, R. A.
Aaron Diamond AIDS Research Center and the Rockefeller University, 455 First Avenue, 7th Floor, New York, NY 10016, USA

Kurth, R.
Paul-Ehrlich-Institute, Paul-Ehrlich-Str. 51-59, 63225 Langen, Germany

Lacey, S. F.
Departement of Surgery, Box 2926, Duke University Medical Center, Durham, NC 27710, USA

Lam, G. K.
Laboratory of Immunoregulation, National Institute of Allergy and Infectious Diseases, National Institutes of Health, 10 Center Drive MSC 1876, Building 10, Room 11B13, Bethesda, MD 20892-1876, USA

Meyaard, L.
Department od Clinical Viro-Immunology, Central Laboratory of the Netherlands
Red Cross Blood Transfusion Service and the Laboratory of Experimental and
Clinical Immunology of the University of Amsterdam, Plesmanlaan 125, 1066 CX
Amsterdam, The Netherlands

Miedema, F.
Department of Human Retrovirology, Academie Medical Centre, Amsterdam,
The Netherlands

Montefiori, D. C.
Departement of Surgery, Box 2926, Duke University Medical Center, Durham,
NC 27710, USA

Norley, S.
Paul-Ehrlich-Institute, Paul-Ehrlich-Str. 51-59, 63225 Langen, Germany

Pantaleo, G.
Laboratory of AIDS Immunopathogenesis, Department of Medicine, Division of
Infectious Diseases, Centre Hospitalier Universitaire Vadois (CHUV), 1011
Lausanne, Switzerland

Paxton, W. A.
Aaron Diamond AIDS Research Center and the Rockefeller University, 455 First
Avenue, 7th Floor, New York, NY 10016, USA

Richman, D. D.
University of California, San Diego, Departement of Medicine and Pathology and
the San Diego Veterans Affairs Medical Center, San Diego, California, USA

Walker, B. D.
AIDS Research Center, Massachusetts General Hospital, Harvard Medical School,
Fruit Street, Boston, MA 02114, USA

Weinhold, K. J.
Departement of Surgery, Box 2926, Duke University Medical Center, Durham,
NC 27710, USA

Introduction: Recent advances in the pathogenesis of human immunodeficiency virus infection

Giuseppe Pantaleo[1], Anthony S. Fauci[2]

[1] Laboratory of AIDS Immunopathogenesis, Department of Medicine, Division of Infectious Diseases, Centre Hospitalier Universitaire Vadois (CHUV), CH-1011 Lausanne, Switzerland
[2] Laboratory of Immunoregulation, National Institute of Allergy and Infectious Diseases, National Institutes of Health, Building 31, 31 Center Drive MSC 2520, Room 7A-03, Bethesda, MD 20892–2520, USA

During the last 5 years, major advances have been made in our understanding of the pathogenesis of human immunodeficiency virus (HIV) disease and in the development of new potent antiviral agents. With regard to HIV pathogenesis, several recent observations have not only changed our perspective of HIV disease, but have been critical for the design of therapeutic strategies. These observations include:

1. The delineation of the virologic and immunologic events associated with primary HIV infection. These studies have provided the basis for understanding the mechanisms of viral persistence and escape despite the presence of a powerful HIV-specific immune response.

2. The development of highly sensitive molecular techniques including polymerase chain reaction (PCR) assays for the determination of HIV RNA in plasma, together with the identification of lymphoid tissue as the primary anatomic site for HIV replication and spreading. These studies have demonstrated that virus replication is active and continuous throughout the entire course of HIV disease, including the variably prolonged period of clinical latency, thus demonstrating that true microbiologic latency does not exist in HIV infection.

3. The characterization of the dynamics of HIV infection. These studies have provided accurate calculations of virus turnover, allowing an appreciation of the extraordinarily high numbers of HIV particles produced daily, and have provided the basis for recent studies that have demonstrated the importance during chronic infection of the magnitude of circulating HIV RNA as a predictor of disease progression.

4. The identification of chemokines with suppressor activity on HIV replication and the discovery of co-receptor molecules for HIV entry.

Delineation of the virologic and immunologic events associated with primary infection is critical for undestanding the pathogenesis of HIV infection. Pantaleo et al. have extensively discussed both the virologic and immunologic events occurring during primary HIV infection. It is now clear that lymphoid tissue represents the primary anatomic site for the initial spreading and dissemination and chronic establishment of HIV infection; furthermore, the peak of viremia detected early during primary infection is the result of systemic dissemination of virus throughout the lymphoid tissues. Rapid changes in distribution of virus lead to the establishment of chronic HIV infection within 2–4 weeks after HIV entry; this is associated with the appearance of trapped virions in the follicular dendritic cell (FDC) network of lymphoid tissue. With regard to immunologic events associated with HIV infection, qualitative differences in the pattern of the immune response have been observed among different HIV-infected individuals; more importantly, these qualitative differences are independent predictors of the subsequent clinical outcome. Furthermore, rapid deletion of HIV-specific cytotoxic CD8$^+$ T cell clones may occur during primary infection and, paradoxically, HIV-specific cytotoxic T cells accumulate in blood rather than the lymph nodes prior to the occurrence of down-regulation of HIV in both blood and lymphoid tissue. This information regarding the early immunologic and virologic events provides new insights into the mechanisms of virus escape from the immune response, and suggests that antiviral therapy should be started as early as possible during primary infection and that the time of initiation of therapy may be crucial for preventing chronic establishment of HIV infection and deletion of HIV-specific cytotoxic T cell clones.

Havlir and Richman have analyzed the role of viral dynamics in the pathogenesis of HIV disease and the implications for antiviral therapy. The number of virus particles produced every day is extraordinarily high (7×10^{10}), and the apparently stable levels of viremia in the plasma result from a dynamic equilibrium between the number of virions and infected cells cleared and the number of newly infected cells that are responsible for the virions that are produced every day. The high levels of viral load throughout the course of infection represent the primary mechanism of HIV disease, and accordingly the levels of viremia are predictors of the clinical course in individuals with chronic HIV infection. These observations further support the need for the initiation of potent combination antiviral therapy, which, by significantly reducing viral load, may prevent loss of CD4$^+$ T cells and emergence of virus mutants; furthermore, such therapy may swing the pendulum from a progressive to a nonprogressive course of HIV disease.

The importance of delineating the complex interaction between HIV and the immune system of the host is underscored by Meyaard and Miedema. Several experimental results clearly indicate that the depletion of CD4$^+$ T cells cannot be explained in vivo by direct HIV-mediated cytopathicity. In this regard, several observations have demonstrated that the increased apoptosis in HIV infection involves both CD4$^+$ and CD8$^+$ T cells, thus indicating that T cell death is the result of a more general immune-based mechanism such as immune activation. Furthermore, the profound immune dysfunction cannot be explained only on the basis of the loss of CD4$^+$ T cells but can be extended to all the components of the immune response. The obvious consequence of this general immune dysfunction involving both immune- competent and incompetent cells is the cytokine dysregulation associated with the different phases of HIV infection. Cytokines play a major role in the modulation of the immune response, and the abnormal patterns of cytokines observed in HIV-infected individuals may significantly influence the development of more effective versus less effective immune responses in the control of virus spreading and replication. Therefore, delineation of the immunopathogenesis of HIV infection is critical for delineating protective versus non-protective immune responses and for the development of immune-based therapeutic strategies.

The role of lymphoid organs as the primary anatomic site for virus spreading and replication during chronic infection is discussed by Cohen et al. HIV replication is persistent throughout HIV infection, and this is certainly the primary mechanism responsible for the progressive destruction of lymphoid tissue architecture. Of interest is the minimal effect on viral load in lymphoid tissue of double therapy with reverse transcriptase inhibitors during chronic infection. These findings indicate that triple combination therapies with more potent antiviral drugs will be needed to down-regulate viral load in lymphoid tissue, and that determination of viral load in these tissues is crucial for the correct evaluation of the effectiveness of antiviral therapy.

A number of factors including the route, magnitude, frequency of exposure, genetics of the host, and ability to generate an effective immune response significantly influence the mechanisms leading to susceptibility as well as resistance to HIV infection. Paxton and Koup have addressed these issues by analyzing the apparent resistance to HIV infection in highly exposed individuals. Major advances in understanding the mechanisms of resistance have led to the demonstration that resistance to HIV infection may result from the lack of expression of the co-receptor (CCR5) for HIV in individuals who are homozygous for a defect in the gene encoding for CCR5 which is the co-receptor for macrophage-tropic strains of HIV. However, since this genetic defect is present in a minor percentage of individuals (1% of Caucasians), this defect may explain resistance to HIV infection only in a minority of multiply exposed individuals. Therefore, it is highly likely that the type of immune response, particularly that generated at the site of exposure, i.e., at the level of the mucosa, plays a major role in the protection against HIV infection.

Among the different components of the immune response that play an important role in the mechanisms of protection against HIV infection and in the control of virus replication, HIV-specific cytotoxic T cells are the effector immune mechanisms that have been most extensively investigated. The experimental data that virus-specific cytotoxic T cells are critical in the protective mechanisms against a number of human viruses such as cytomegalovirus, Epstein-Barr virus, hepatitis virus, and the murine lymphocytic choriomeningitis virus are highly convincing. In contrast, the protective role of HIV-specific cytotoxic T cells is still largely debated. Jassoy and Walker, however, provide clear evidence that these cells are certainly important in the control of HIV infection. In support of this hypothesis, they also demonstrate that virus-specific cytotoxic T cells are mostly responsible for the antiviral suppressor activity mediated by a CD8$^+$ T cell-derived soluble factor.

In this regard, the CD8$^+$ T cell-derived anti-HIV suppressor factor is extensively analyzed by Greenberg et al. Although these authors provide additional experimental data that this suppressor activity is mediated by the β-chemokines, they agree with other investigators that other still-unidentified factors are likely to be responsible for the CD8$^+$ T cell suppressor activity. Furthemore, the implications of these recent findings for the development of new immune-based therapeutic and preventive strategies are also examined.

The role of complement and Fc receptors in the pathogenesis of HIV infection is examined by Montefiori. He provides evidence that the formation of complexes between HIV and complement may lead to more efficient virus entry, to the propagation of infection over time by the establishment of a virus reservoir in the FDC network, and to the disruption of B cell function. Furthermore, formation of complexes between HIV particles and immunoglobulins may enhance HIV infection of FcR$^+$ cells such as macrophages.

Finally, Norley and Kurth have underscored the importance of studying the various SIV/primate animal models for dissecting the pathogenic events leading to AIDS. We are hopeful that this volume will provide a useful summary of the recent advances in the pathogenesis of HIV disease.

Virologic and immunologic events in primary HIV infection

Guiseppe Pantaleo[1], Cecilia Graziosi[1], Anthony S. Fauci[2]

[1]Laboratory of AIDS Immunopathogenesis, Department of Internal Medicine, Division of Infectious Diseases, Centre Hospitalier Universitaire Vaudois (CHUV), CH-1011 Lausanne, Switzerland
[2]Laboratory of Immunoregulation, National Institute of Allergy and Infectious Diseases, National Institutes of Health, Building 31, 31 Center Drive MSC 2520, Room 7A-03, MD 20892-2520, USA

Introduction

It is thought that a significant percentage (50–70%) of human immunodeficiency virus (HIV)-infected individuals experience a clinical syndrome of variable severity during primary infection. The symptoms are non specific, typical of a flu-like syndrome [7, 10, 47], and include fever, sore throat, nausea, diarrhea, skin rash, myalgia, lymphadenopathy, and only rarely meningitis. However, due to the lack of specificity and to the variable severity of the clinical syndrome, hospitalization or medical intervention is required in only a minority of cases, and thus primary infection usually goes unnoticed.

Over the past 5 years, major advances have been made in the delineation of the virologic and immunologic events associated with primary infection; analysis of these events has been performed in individuals experiencing an acute clinical syndrome. Although the possibility that virologic and immunologic events associated with primary infection may be substantially different in asymptomatic individuals, it is generally accepted that those events that are described for symptomatic individuals reflect fairly accurately the sequelae of pathogenic events occurring in asymptomatic individuals. It is, however, appropriate to point out that it is possible that important differences may exist between the two groups. These may include different levels of initial peak viremia as well as qualitative differences in the primary virus-specific immune response. Further studies are necessary to delineate the influence of these potential differences on the control of virus spreading and replication, and on the clinical outcome of HIV infection.

Distribution of HIV in different lymphoid compartments

Kinetic studies of the distribution of HIV/simian immunodeficiency virus (SIV) in different lymphoid compartments have led to the delineation of the sequelae of virologic events associated with primary infection. The distribution of HIV/SIV in lymph nodes has been investigated by performing either sequential lymph node biopsies, i.e., longitudinal analysis, in monkeys inoculated with SIV [30, 34, 37], or single lymph node biopsies in different HIV-infected individuals either during primary infection or within 12 months of seroconversion, i.e., cross-sectional analysis (Pantaleo et al., unpublished observations). SIV may be detected in lymph node biopsy samples as early as 5 days post-inoculation [30, 37]. At this time during primary infection, SIV is present in lymph nodes almost exclusively in the form of numerous individual cells expressing viral RNA, as clearly demonstrated by in situ hybridization. Two findings indicate that lymph nodes are the primary anatomic sites for the initial establishment of infection: the peak number of virus-expressing cells is observed as early as day 7 post-inoculation [30, 37]; and the peak number of virus-expressing cells in the lymph node is found concomitant with and/or precedes the peak viremia in the blood [30, 37]. The appearance of virus trapped in the follicular dendritic cell (FDC) network of lymph node germinal centers represents the dominant form of virus present in lymph nodes after the transition to the chronic phase of infection. Virus trapping is associated with a dramatic decrease in the number of individual cells expressing viral RNA [30, 34, 37]. The rapid decrease in individual cells expressing virus is probably the result of the emergence of a virus-specific immune response; in particular, virus-specific cytotoxic T cells are responsible for the elimination of productively infected cells. Virus trapped in the FDC network is complexed with immunoglobulin (Ig) and complement (C′), and the binding of these complexes on the extracellular surface of FDCs occurs through C′ receptors expressed on the surface of FDCs [2, 15-17, 33, 35, 43, 44]. Of note is the observation that trapped virus is highly infectious despite the fact that it is complexed with Ig and C′ [21].

Cross-sectional analyses of lymph node biopsy specimens from HIV-infected individuals obtained during primary infection and early after seroconversion have confirmed that the kinetics of virus distribution in lymph nodes observed in the SIV model of acute infection are valid for HIV infection (Pantaleo et al., unpublished observations). Furthermore, in both SIV and HIV infections the switch over time from individual virus-expressing cells to trapped virus in the FDC network of lymph node germinal centers reflects the transition from the acute to the chronic phase of SIV/HIV infection. In this regard, the progressive increase of virus trapping during primary infection is associated with down-regulation of plasma viremia and resolution of the acute clinical syndrome.

Primary HIV-specific immune response

Both HIV-specific humoral and cell-mediated immune responses are detected very early during primary infection [4, 7, 10, 26, 29, 36, 40]. These immune responses play a critical role in the initial down-regulation of virus replication and in the control of virus spreading over time. The different components of the HIV-specific immune response include: (a) HIV-specific cytotoxicity, (b) cytokine responses, and (c) HIV-specific antibody response.

Cell-mediated immune response

HIV-specific cell-mediated immune responses are detected very early during primary infection and likely precede the virus-specific humoral response [4, 26, 36, 40]. A major component of the HIV-specific cell-mediated immune response is represented by large expansions of CD8$^+$ T lymphocytes [36]. During the initial weeks of infection the absolute number of circulating CD8$^+$ T lymphocytes may increase up to 20-fold above the normal range (200–600/μl blood; Pantaleo et al., unpublished observations). Analysis of the T cell receptor (TCR) repertoire has demonstrated that these large increases in CD8$^+$ T cells reflect mono-oligoclonal expansions of these cells during primary infection [36]. In contrast, a significant drop in the absolute number of circulating CD4$^+$ T lymphocytes is observed, and CD4$^+$ T cell-mediated functions are severely depressed. CD8$^+$ T lymphocytes may contribute to the suppression of virus replication by two mechanisms: HIV-specific cytotoxicity [4, 26, 36, 40], and suppression by soluble factors [27]. It has been demonstrated that these activities mediated by CD8$^+$ T lymphocytes are detected very early during primary infection [4, 26, 27, 36, 40]. Virus-specific cytotoxic T lymphocytes (CTL) can be detected as early as 5 days following initial infection, as demonstrated in the SIV model of acute infection [40]. In addition, the appearance of HIV-specific CTL generally coincides with the down-regulation of viremia [26]. HIV-specific CTL are directed against both structural (gag and env) and regulatory (tat and rev) proteins of HIV, and their precursor frequency is high, i.e., HIV-specific CTL are readily detected in blood, and their frequency may vary significantly, ranging from 1:100 to 1:10,000 among different subjects ([26] and Pantaleo et al., unpublished observations). HIV suppressor activity mediated by soluble factors derived from CD8$^+$ T cells is also detected in patients with primary infection [27]. The importance of the initial virus-specific CD8$^+$ T cell-mediated response in the down-regulation of virus replication is strongly supported by the observation that a delay in the appearance of HIV-specific CTL is generally associated with a prolonged acute viral syndrome and the persistence of high levels of viremia [26].

Cytokine response

The pattern of cytokine response during primary HIV infection has been recently studied [19]. Analysis of the expression of a panel of cytokines including interleukin (IL)-2, IL-4, IL-6, IL-10, tumor necrosis factor-α (TNF-α), and interferon-γ (INF-γ) has been performed on peripheral blood mononuclear cell samples collected at different time points during primary infection and after the transition to the chronic phase of infection. This longitudinal analysis demonstrated an early peak in the expression of IFN-γ in a significant percentage (up to 50%) of the patients studied [19]. Substantial expression of IL-10 and TNF-α was observed in all patients analyzed [19]. However, in contrast to IFN-γ, expression of these cytokines increased progressively during the transition from the acute to the chronic phase of infection. IL-2 and IL-4 expression was barely detected in blood mononuclear cells, and IL-6 expression was observed only in a minority of patients; when IL-6 was detected, a peak in expression was observed after the transition to the chronic phase of infection [19]. This pattern of cytokine expression was correlated with the other components of the primary immune response to HIV. The peak in expression of IFN-γ coincided with the expansion of

CD8$^+$ T lymphocytes and, in particular, with the peak in the expression of certain CD8$^+$ Vβ T cell subsets (see below), which represents a major component of the primary immune response to HIV [19, 30]. Although it is unclear whether IFN-γ has any role in the initial control of HIV spreading and replication, several observations indicate that cytokines may have a fundamental role in the virus-specific immune response. In this regard, it has recently been shown that IFN-γ and TNF-α, but not virus-specific CTL, mediate the viricidal effect in hepatitis B virus infection [20]. Furthermore, the expanded CD8$^+$ T lymphocytes may secrete a series of soluble factors in addition to IFN-γ, i.e., β-chemokines (RANTES, MIP-1α and MIP-1β) [8], that are the natural ligands for the coreceptor (CCR5) of M-tropic strains of HIV [1, 6, 11, 13, 14], and thus potentially mediate suppression of virus spreading and replication by preventing infection of the target cells of HIV. Thus, cytokines and chemokines are an important component of the primary immune response in several virus infections, and may play a major role in their initial control.

Humoral response

The role of the HIV-specific humoral immune response in the down-regulation of virus replication during primary infection has been debated. Although anti-HIV antibodies are barely detected in the early stages of primary infection, high titers of antibodies specific for a variety of HIV proteins are detected at the time of the peak and subsequent down-regulation of viremia [7, 10 , 29, 47]. However, neutralizing antibodies that are felt to represent the protective component of the HIV-specific humoral immune response are generally not detected during primary infection and appear late after down-regulation of viremia and when the transition to the chronic phase of infection has already occurred [26]. Therefore, it is unlikely that the HIV-specific humoral immune response plays any role in limiting the spread of HIV during the early stages of infection. This, however, does not exclude the possibility that HIV antibodies may contribute to the down-regulation of viremia by a mechanical mechanism. In fact, it is conceivable that a proportion of the HIV antibodies produced during primary infection have C$'$ binding activity, and thus may mediate the formation of immune complexes formed by antibody plus HIV plus C$'$. These immune complexes may remain trapped either in the FDC network (FDCs express C$'$ receptors) or in the reticuloendothelial system (see above). Therefore, these observations indicate an important role of the HIV-specific humoral response in the removal of virus particles from the circulation and in mediating virus trapping in the FDC network of lymph node germinal centers [30, 37].

Mechanisms of virus escape from the immune response

Both virologic and immunologic mechanisms may potentially contribute to HIV escape from the immune response during primary infection [31]. Analysis and identification of these mechanisms are of extreme importance in understanding why HIV is able to persist and induce chronic infection despite the fact that a vigorous virus-specific immune response is detected very early during primary infection. Here, we will discuss briefly a series of mechanisms which when taken individually may not explain the failure of the immune response to eliminate HIV; however, when taken

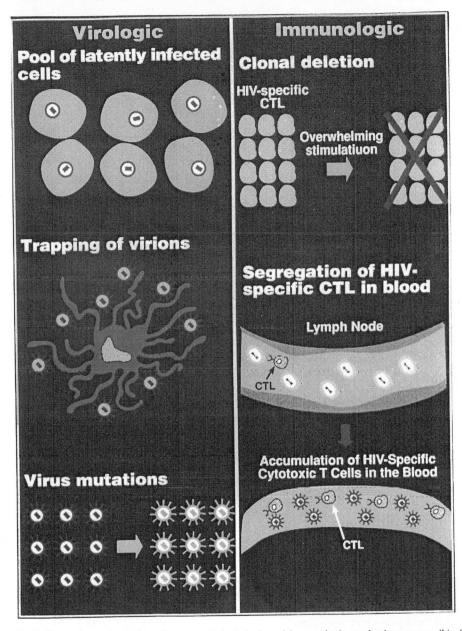

Fig. 1. Schematic representation of the potential virologic and immunologic mechanisms responsibie for virus escape from the immune response during primary HIV infection

together they may tilt the delicate balance between the host immune response and virus in favor of virus spreading and replication, thus promoting the persistence of HIV and progression to chronic infection.

Several virologic mechanisms may contribute substantially to virus escape from the immune response during primary infection (Fig. 1). These include: (a) generation of a large pool of latently infected cells (i.e., containing HIV provirus DNA) [18]; (b) trapping of virions in the FDC network of lymph node germinal centers [30, 37]; and (c) changes in virus phenotype and genotype [28, 39].

A comparison of the kinetics of changes in the levels of plasma viremia and the number of HIV DNA copies in peripheral blood mononuclear cells has shown a discrepancy between the dramatic down-regulation of viremia and the minimal changes in the number of HIV DNA copies in blood mononuclear cells during the transition from the acute to the chronic phase of infection [18]. Since most latently infected cells contain defective virus [9], it is unlikely that this mechanism significantly influences the course of HIV disease. However, the pool of latently infected cells may have an important role in the propagation of HIV infection under certain circumstances. For example, a rapid increase in the levels of viremia and a substantial increment in the percentage of activated CD4$^+$ T lymphocytes that are the major target of HIV have been observed during the course of opportunistic infections in HIV-infected individuals [12, 22-24, 48]. Furthermore, although certain anti-retroviral drugs may potently suppress virus replication, they have little, if any, effect on the pool of latently infected cells.

Trapping of virus particles in the FDC network of lymph node germinal centers is certainly an important mechanism of both virus escape from the immune response and propagation of infection over time. It has been shown recently that these trapped virions are infectious despite the fact that they are coupled with antibody and C' [21]. A likely scenario is that these trapped virions represent a continuous source of virus for de novo infection of suceptible target cells; furthermore, by inducing a chronic immune stimulation, they maintain a constant pool of activated CD4$^+$ T cells that can support high levels of virus replication.

Finally, changes in virus genotype and phenotype may also represent important mechanisms of virus escape from the immune response. However, it is likely that this mechanism plays a major role during chronic infection rather than in primary infection. The loss of virus-specific cytotoxic activity may result from either variations in the viral epitopes recognized by CTL [39] or from naturally occurring mutations within the CTL epitope that may inhibit T cell effector function by acting as antagonists [28]. The appearance of syncytium-inducing (SI) strains of HIV is generally associated with rapid progression of HIV disease [3, 25, 41, 42, 45, 46]. It is conceivable that the immune response is poorly effective in the control of SI strains of HIV that have a high replicating capability.

A series of immunologic mechanisms have been recently identified during primary infection that may significantly contribute to tilting the balance towards virus spreading and replication, thus promoting persistence of HIV (Fig. 1). These include: (a) a qualitatively inadequate immune response; (b) deletion of expanded HIV-specific CTL clones; and (c) accumulation of HIV-specific CTLs away from the primary site of virus spreading and replication.

The analysis of standard parameters of the immune response such as cytotoxic activity and antibody response have failed to provide significant insight into the evolution of effective immune responses to HIV infection [30]. A more precise analysis of the immune response by delineation of the kinetics of changes in the TCR repertoire have clearly demonstrated qualitative differences in the primary immune response to HIV among different individuals. In particular, it has been shown that individuals who respond to HIV with a restricted (mostly involving one Vβ family) TCR repertoire generally experience a rapid course of HIV infection with progression to AIDS within 2-4 years. In contrast, those individuals who respond with a broad (multiple $V\beta$ families) TCR repertoire generally have slow progression of HIV disease [38]. Therefore, qualitative differences in the primary immune response to HIV may be associated with inadequate protection against disease progression.

Rapid deletion of HIV-specific cytotoxic $CD8^+$ T cell clones have been observed during primary infection ([31] and Pantaleo et al., unpublished observations). Generally, these rapidly deleted virus-specific clones are contained in the $CD8^+$ $V\beta$ T cell subsets that undergo major expansions. In this regard, deletion of HIV-specific cytotoxic T cell clones may represent the major mechanism of the rapid collapse of the immune response in those individuals who respond with a restricted TCR repertoire. Furthermore, it is conceivable that the high levels of HIV associated with primary infection play an important role in the deletion phenomenon. It is also important that lymphoid tissue, which is the anatomic site in which an immune response is generated, is also the primary site for virus spreading and replication. Based on these observations, it is likely that during primary infection there is an overwhelming stimulation of the small number of precursor cells specific for a given HIV antigen as a result of exceptionally high levels of antigen and of its concentration in the same anatomic compartment (lymphoid tissue) in which immune the response is generated.

Finally, comparative analysis of the frequencies of in vivo HIV-specific CTL and of CTL precursors has demonstrated a greater accumulation of cytotoxic T cells in peripheral blood as compared to lymph node ([31] and Pantaleo et al., unpublished observations). This observation is particularly important since at the time of the accumulation of CTL in blood, plasma viremia has not been effectively curtailed and active virus replication is detected in lymph nodes.

Conclusions

Lymphoid tissue represents the primary anatomic site for virus spreading, replication and initial establishment of HIV infection. The burst of viremia associated with primary HIV infection results in the systemic dissemination of virus throughout the lymphoid tissue. Despite the appearance of a vigorous immune response, HIV is not completely eliminated, but is only partially controlled. The lack of elimination of HIV is likely the result of a series of virologic and immunologic mechanisms that are operative at the time of primary infection. These mechanisms play a major role in virus escape from the immune response and, in particular, certain immunologic mechanisms may substantially influence the course of HIV infection. These observations provide further evidence that the initial interaction and delicate balance between the virus and the immune system of the host are critical for the subsequent outcome of the infection, i.e., elimination or persistence of virus.

References

1. Alkhatib G, Combardiere C, Broder CC, Feng Y, Kennedy PE, Murphy P, Berger E (1996) CC CKR5: a RANTES, MIP-1α, MIP-1β receptor as a fusion cofactor for macrophage-tropic HIV-1. Science 272:1955
2. Armstrong JA, Dawkins RL, Horne R (1985) Retroviral infection of accessory cells and the immunological paradox in AIDS. Immunol Today 6:121

3. Asjo B, Sharma UK, Morfeldt-Manson L, Magnusson A (1990) Naturally occurring HIV-1 isolates with differences in replicative capacity are distinguished by in situ hybridization of infected cells. AIDS Res Hum Retroviruses 6:1177

4. Borrow P, Lewicki H, Hahn BH, Shaw GM, Oldstone MB (1994) CTL activity associated with control of viremia in primary HIV-1 infection. J Virol 68:6103

5. Reference deleted

6. Choe H, Farzan M, Sun Y, Sullivan N, Rollins B, Ponath PD, Wu L, Mackay CR, LaRosa G, Newman W, Gerard N, Gerard C, Sodroski J (1996) The β-chemokine receptors CCR3 and CCR5 facilitate infection by primary HIV-1 isolates. Cell 85:1135

7. Clark SJ, Saag MS, Decker WD, Campbell-Hill S, Roberson JL, Veldkamp PJ, Kappes JC, Hahn BH, Shaw GM (1991) High titers of cytopathic virus in plasma of patients with symptomatic primary HIV-1 infection. N Engl J Med 324:954

8. Cocchi F, DeVico AL, Garzino-Demo A, Ayra SK, Gallo RC, Lusso P (1996) Identification of RANTES, MIP-1α, and MIP-1β as the major HIV-suppressive factors produced by CD8$^+$ T cells. Science 270:1811

9. Coffin JM (1995) HIV population dynamics in vivo: implications for genetic variation, pathogenesis, and therapy Science 267:483

10. Daar ES, Moudgil T, Meyer RD, Ho DD (1991) Transient high levels of viremia in patients with primary human immunodeficiency virus type 1 infection. N Engl J Med 324:961

11. Deng H, Liu R, Ellmeier W, Choe W, Nutmaz D, Burkhart M, Di Marzio P, Marmon S, Sutton RE, Hill CM, Davis CB, Peiper SC, Schall TJ, Littman DR, Laudau NR (1996) Identification of a major co-receptor for primary isolates of HIV-1. Nature 381:661

12. Denis M, Ghadirian E (1994) *Mycobacterium avium* infection in HIV-1-infected subjects increases monokine secretion and is associated with enhanced viral load and diminished immune response to viral antigens. Clin Exp Immunol 97:76-82

13. Doranz BJ, Rucker J, Yi Y, Smyth RJ, Samson M, Peiper SC, Parmentier M, Collman RG, Doms RW (1996) A dual-tropic primary HIV-1 isolate that uses fusin and the b-chemokine receptors CKR-5, CKR-3, and CKR-2b as fusion cofactors. Cell 85:1149

14. Dragic T, Litwin V, Allaway GP, Martin SR, Huang Y, Nagashima KA, Cayanan C, Maddon PJ, Koup R, Moore JP, Paxton WA (1996) HIV-1 entry into CD4$^+$ cells is mediated by the chemokine receptor CC-CKR-5. Nature 381:667

15. Embretson J, Zupancic M, Ribas JL, Burke A, Tenner-Racz K, Haase AT (1993) Massive covert infection of helper T lymphocytes and macrophages by HIV during the incubation period of AIDS. Nature 362:359

16. Emilie D, Peuchmaur M, Maillot M, Crevon M, Brousse N, Delfraissy J, Dormont J, Galanaud P (1990) Production of interleukins in human immunodeficiency virus-1-replicating lymph nodes. J Clin Invest 86:148

17. Fox CH, Tenner-Racz K, Racz P, Firpo A, Pizzo PA, Fauci AS (1991) Lymphoid germinal centers are reservoirs of human immunodeficiency virus type 1 RNA. J Infect Dis 164:1051

18. Graziosi C, Pantaleo G, Butini L, Demarest JF, Saag MS, Shaw GM, Fauci AS (1993) Kinetics of HIV DNA and RNA synthesis during primary HIV-1 infection. Proc Natl Acad Sci USA 90:6505

19. Graziosi C, Gantt KR, Vaccarezza M, Demarest JF, Daucher MB, Saag MS, Shaw GM, Quinn TC, Cohen OJ, Welbon C, Pantaleo G, Fauci AS (1996) Kinetics of cytokine expression during primary human immunodeficiency virus type 1 (HIV-1) infection. Proc Natl Acad Sci USA, 93:4386

20. Guidotti LG, Ishikawa T, Hobbs MV, Matzke B, Scrieber, Chisari FV (1996) Intracellular inactivation of the hepatitis B virus by cytotoxic T lymphocytes. Immunity 4:25

21. Health SL, Tew JG, Szakal AK, Burton GF (1995) Follicular dendritic cells and human immunodeficiency virus. Nature 377:740

22. Heng MCY, Heng SY, Allen SG (1994) Co-infection and synergy of human immunodeficiency virus-1 and herpes simplex virus-1. Lancet 343:255

23. Ho DD (1992) HIV-1 viraemia and influenza. Lancet 339:1549

24. Israel-Biet D, Cadranel J, Even P (1993) Human immunodeficiency virus production by alveolar lymphocytes is increased during *Pneumocystis carinii* pneumonia. Am Rev Respir Dis 148:1308

25. Koot M, Keet IP, Vos AH, deGoede RE, Roos MT, Coutinho RA, Miedema F, Schellekens PT, Tersmette M (1993) Prognostic value of HIV-1 syncytium-inducing phenotype for rate of CD4$^+$ cell depletion and progression to AIDS. Ann Intern Med 118:681

26. Koup RA, Safrit JT, Cao Y, Andrews CA, McLeod G, Ho DD (1994) Temporal association of cellular immune responses with the initial control of viremia in primary human immunodeficiency virus type 1 syndrome. J Virol 68:4650
27. Mackewicz CF, Ortega HW, Levy JA (1991) CD8+ cell anti-HIV activity correlates with the clinical state of the infected individuals. J Clin Invest 87:1462
28. Meier UC, Klenerman P, Griffin P, James W, Koppe B, Larder B, McMichael A, Phillips R (1995) Cytotoxic T lymphocyte lysis inhibited by viable HIV mutants. Science 270:1360
29. Moore JP, Cao Y, Ho DD, Koup RA (1994) Development of the anti-gp120 antibody response during seroconversion to human immunodeficiency virus type 1. J Virol 68:5142
30. Pantaleo G, Fauci AS (1995) New concepts in the immunopathogenesis of HIV infection. Annu Rev Immunol 13:487
31. Pantaleo G, Fauci AS (1996) Immunopathogenesis of HIV infection. Annu Rev Microbiol 50:825
32. Pantaleo G, Graziosi C, Butini L, Pizzo PA, Schnittman SM, Kotler DP, Fauci AS (1991) Lymphoid organs function as major reservoirs for human immunodeficiency virus. Proc Natl Acad Sci USA 88:9838
33. Pantaleo G, Graziosi C, Demarest JF, Butini L, Montroni M, Fox CH, Orenstein JM, Kotler DP, Fauci AS (1993) HIV infection is active and progressive in lymphoid tissue during the clinically latent stage of disease. Nature 362:355
34. Pantaleo G, Graziosi C, Fauci AS (1993) The role of lymphoid organs in the pathogenesis of HIV infection. Semin Immunol 5:157
35. Pantaleo G, Graziosi C, Fauci AS (1993) The role of lymphoid organs in the immunopathogenesis of HIV infection. AIDS 7:S19
36. Pantaleo G, Demarest JF, Soudeyns H, Graziosi C, Denis F, Saag M, Shaw GM, Sekaly RP, Fauci AS (1994) Major expansion of CD8+ T cells with a predominant Vβ usage during the primary immune response of HIV. Nature 370:463
37. Pantaleo G, Graziosi C, Demarest JF, Cohen OJ, Vaccarezza M, Muro-Cacho C, Fauci AS (1994) Role of lymphoid organs in the pathogenesis of human immunodeficiency virus (HIV) infection. Immunol Rev 140:105
38. Pantaleo G, Demarest JF, Schacker T, Vaccarezza M, Cohen OJ, Daucher MB, Graziosi C, Schnittman SM, Quinn TC, Shaw GM, Perrin L, Tambussi G, Lazzarin A, Sekaly RP, Soudeyns H, Corey L, Fauci AS (1997) The qualitative nature of the primary immune response to HIV infection is a prognosticator of disease progression independent of the initial level of plasma viremia. Proc Natl Acad Sci USA 94:254
39. Philips RE, Rowland-Jones S, Nixon DF, Gotch FM, Edwards JP, Ogunlesi AO, Elvin JG, Rothbard JA, Bangham CR, Rizza CR, McMichael A (1991) Human immunodeficiency virus genetic variation that can escape cytotoxic T cell recognition. Nature 354:453
40. Reimann KA, Tenner-Racz K, Racz P, Montefiori DC, Yasutomi Y, Letvin NL (1994). Immunopathogenic events in acute infection of Rhesus monkeys with simian immunodeficiency virus of Macaques. J Virol 68:2362
41. Schellekens PT, Tersmette M, Roos MT, Keet RP, Wolf F de, Coutinho RA, Miedema F (1992) Biphasic rate of CD4+ cell count decline during progression to AIDS correlates with HIV-1 phenotype. AIDS 6:665
42. Schuitemaker H, Koot M, Koostra NA, Dercksen MW, Goede REY de, Steenwijk RP van, Lange JM, Schattenkerk JK, Miedema F, Tersmette M (1992) Biological phenotype of human immunodeficiency virus type 1 clones at different stages of infection: progression of disease is associated with a shift from monocytotropic to T-cell-tropic virus population. J Virol 66:1354
43. Spiegel H, Herbst H, Niedobitek G, Foss HD, Stein H (1992) Follicular dendritic cells are a major reservoir for human immunodeficiency virus type 1 in lymphoid tissues facilitating infection of CD4+ T-helper cells. Am J Pathol 140:15
44. Tenner-Racz K, Racz P, Dietrich M, Karin P (1985) Altered follicular dendritic cells and virus-like particles in AIDS and AIDS related lymphadenopathy. Lancet I:105

45. Tersmette M, Goede RE de, Al BJ, Winkel IN, Gruters RA, Cuypers HT, Huisman HG, Miedema F
    (1988) Differential syncytium-inducing capacity of human immunodeficiency virus isolates: frequent
    detection of syncytium-inducing isolates in patients with acquired immunodeficiency syndrome (AIDS)
    and AIDS-related complex. J Virol 62:2026
46. Tersmette M, Gruters RA, Wolf F de, Goede RE de, Lange JM, Schellekens PT, Goudsmit J, Huisman
    HG, Miedema F (1989) Evidence for a role of virulent human immunodeficiency virus (HIV) variants
    in the pathogenesis of acquired immunodeficiency syndrome: sudies on sequential HIV isolates. J Virol
    63:2118
47. Tindall B, Cooper DA (1991) Primary HIV infection: host responses and intervention strategies. AIDS
    5:1
48. Zhang Y, Nakata K, Weiden M, Rom WN (1995) *Mycobacterium tuberculosis* enhances human im-
    munodeficiency virus-1 replication by transcriptional activation at the long terminal repeat. J Clin
    Invest 95:2324

The role of viral dynamics in the pathogenesis of HIV disease and implications for antiviral therapy

Diane V. Havlir, Douglas D. Richman

University of California, San Diego, Departments of Medicine and Pathology and the San Diego Veterans Affairs Medical Center, San Diego, California

Introduction

Recent insights into the dynamics of human immunodeficiency virus (HIV) replication have increased our understanding of the pathogenesis of HIV disease [9, 25]. Throughout the course of HIV disease, including the period of clinical latency, an extraordinary number of virus particles are produced daily leading to the gradual destruction and depletion of CD4 T lymphocytes [31, 74]. The magnitude of circulating HIV RNA is an important predictor of the pace of immunologic deterioration and clinical disease progression which varies by more than 10 years among individuals [28, 44]. Antiretroviral therapy reduces HIV replication but the rapid turnover of virus provides ample opportunity for drug-resistant mutants to emerge [57]. Current therapeutic strategies include the use of multiple drugs directed at different targets of the HIV life cycle to maximize the magnitude and durability of virus suppression and minimize the emergence of escape mutants.

Primary infection and clinical latency

Primary infection with HIV is characterized by a rapid increase in viral titers with simultaneous widespread dissemination of virus throughout the lymphatic tissues [8, 15]. Limited data indicate that HIV RNA concentrations reach peak levels of 10^5–10^8 copies/ml of plasma within weeks after initial infection. One hundred to ten thousand infectious units of HIV can be detected per million peripheral blood mononuclear cells and precede the detection of HIV antibodies by standard enzyme immunoassays.

Correspondence to: Diane Havlir, UCSD Treatment Center, 2760 Fifth Avenue, Ste. 300, San Diego, CA 92103, USA

Between one third and two thirds of individuals have been estimated to develop a clinical syndrome (fever, headache, myalgia, sore throat, and rash) during this early period of virus replication which is self limited and typically resolves within 12 weeks of primary infection.

Although systematic studies which capture frequent measures of viral load have not been performed in large numbers of individuals during primary infection, it appears that there is variability in the peak titers as well as the magnitude of steady-state levels of HIV in the plasma which are established between 6 and 12 months of infection. These steady-state levels correlate strongly with the rate of clinically apparent HIV disease progression [33, 43, 65]. HIV seroconverters who exhibit the classical clinical symptoms of primary infection also appear to have a higher risk for more rapid HIV disease progression [27]. The characterization of these early events is of utmost importance in understanding the pathogenesis of HIV but has been hampered by difficulty in the early identification of HIV seroconverters, particularly those who are asymptomatic.

The decline of HIV titers in the plasma and peripheral blood mononuclear cells at the termination of the primary infection has been attributed to the host immune response. Virus-specific cytotoxic T lymphocytes may play a critical role; their appearance is temporally associated with the decline in viral burden [37]. Presumably, these cells could mediate clearance of HIV-infected cells. While neutralizing antibodies may also play a role in controlling the initial burst of viral replication, they generally appear well after the decline in viral burden, calling into question their role in control of early viral replication.

A model of viral population dynamics raises an alternative hypothesis to explain the rapid decline of virus at the end of primary infection [56]. In this model, the rapid rise in viral titers corresponds to rapid replication of HIV in an initially unlimited supply of uninfected susceptible cells. The reduction in virus concentration observed during the first weeks after infection can be entirely attributed to the exhaustion of permissive host cells. A quasi-steady state is then reached in which the clearance of virus and infected cells is constant and balanced by a constant rate of virus production, which is dependent upon the generation of a steady rate of new permissive host cells. This model predicts that virus levels are determined by levels of permissive host cells, like activated CD4 T lymphocytes, and that an increased rate of clearance of infected cells, such as might be produced by an immunologic response, is not necessary to predict the decline in viral burden following primary infection. This hypothesis implies that the immune response is a consequence of HIV replication and not a cause of its control.

Acute infection with HIV may result from exposure to a known source or donor infected with a complex mixture of genetic variants of HIV; however, a single monoclonal or genetically homogeneous population typically dominates in primary infection [17, 79, 82]. Whether selection occurs at the time of transmission or early during propagation in the host is not known. Shortly after primary infection genetic variation is readily detected (independent of antiretroviral therapy). Evolution of new HIV variants within an infected individual, with "escape" from immunologic control, has been put forth as one explanation for declines of CD4 cell counts and increases in viral burden. One recent study challenges this hypothesis, however, demonstrating that HIV-infected individuals who experience rapid disease progression harbor less genetic variants than clinically stable patients [80]. Moreover, discordance between circulating strains and those in the central nervous system is also observed [20, 76, 81].

After primary infection, clinical symptoms associated with HIV disease are absent and viral markers such as p24 antigen are undetectable. This observation led to the early erroneous conclusion that during this time period of clinical "latency" the virus was also latent. Inconsistent with the concept of "viral latency" were the reports that HIV could be cultured from spinal fluid and identified in the brain [32, 68, 77]. Elegant in situ hybridization studies which demonstrated that large numbers of CD4 lymphocytes and macrophages are HIV-infected definitively refuted that concept of viral latency [3, 21, 51, 71]. HIV is trapped as antibody complexes in the germinal centers of the lymph nodes by the processes of follicular dendritic cells [1, 4, 41, 51, 70, 71]. As many as one-third of CD4 cells in the lymph node and in the blood have detectable HIV DNA, although many genomes have defective replicative capacity [2, 21, 53]. Active replication as measured by HIV RNA expression is present in only 0.1–1% of cells but the large reservoir of uninfected cells is sufficient to generate new rounds of replication and produce a gradually increasing viral burden [21, 53]. Early in clinical latency, viral replication may be five to ten times greater in the lymph tissue compared to the periphery [21, 51, 67].

Quantitative polymerase chain reaction (PCR)-based assays, which are now commercially available, detect HIV RNA during all stages of disease in untreated patients, including this period of clinical latency [46, 73]. Quantitation of HIV RNA with branched chain amplification methodology yields results concordant with PCR methodology but has a less sensitive limit of detection of (10^3 copies/ml) [19]. Similar to culturable titers of HIV, levels of HIV RNA are inversely proportional to CD4 cell counts and HIV disease stage when large numbers of patients are analyzed [12, 30, 63]. It is important to note, however, that a remarkable degree of variability (as much as 1000 fold) is observed among individuals for any given CD4 cell counts. The sensitivity, dynamic range of the HIV RNA assay (10^2–10^6), and ability to measure levels in properly stored specimens have permitted pivotal insights into viral dynamics and the natural history of HIV disease.

Recently completed and ongoing studies suggest that 6–12 months after primary infection, a "set point" HIV RNA level is established which is highly predictive of HIV disease progression [18, 43] (Fig. 1). A small minority of patients whose viral burden remains at high levels after primary infection exhibit a rapid decline in CD4 cell counts and development of opportunistic infections [47]. Another small subset of infected patients maintain low levels of circulating HIV RNA ($< 10^3$ copies/ml plasma) for up to a decade or more [5, 52]. Virus with *nef* deletions and impaired replicative capacity has been isolated from a few of these "long-term nonprogressors" but in the remainder, the explanation for the delayed progression has not been explained [5, 36]. In the majority of patients, HIV RNA levels gradually increase and CD4 cell counts decrease over a period of years. Even a single measurement of HIV RNA is a powerful predictor of subsequent disease course. In a recent study of 181 HIV-infected patients followed over a period of 10 years, HIV RNA levels were independent and more powerful predictors of disease progression than CD4 cell counts [44]. For example, in patients with CD4 cell counts greater than 500 and HIV RNA levels exceeding 10 900 copies/ml plasma, 50% of subjects died within 6 years of observation as opposed to 5% of patients with similar CD4 cell counts and HIV RNA levels below this threshold.

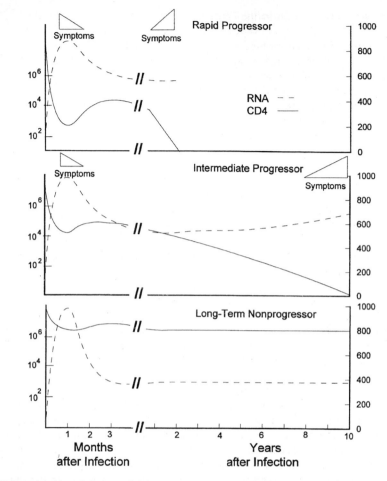

Fig. 1. Schematic of human immunodeficiency virus (HIV) type 1 RNA levels and CD4+ lymphocytes during the course of infection. *Top* Patients rapidly developing clinical symptoms. *Middle* Patients developing clinical disease after 8–10 years. *Bottom* Patients remaining asymptomatic for more than 10 years. The initial burst of virus replication with primary infection is dampened either by the host's immune response or by exhaustion of permissive host cells. Within 6–12 months, each patient appears to establish a steady-state set point for plasma HIV RNA that is highly predictive of subsequent clinical course. Most patients are intermediate progressors. Long-term nonprogressors have low numbers of HIV RNA copies and CD4 cell counts close to the normal range that can remain stable for a decade or more. Great variability in HIV RNA levels exists within these three classifications, and other factors, such as virus phenotype, are independent predictors of outcome. (Figure reproduced with permission from the American College of Physicians [25])

Viral dynamics

The availability of quantitative assays for HIV RNA permits the rapid and precise assessment viral burden in the plasma. Over a period of months, HIV RNA levels remain relatively stable in most patients in the absence of treatment or antigenic stimulation [78]. Vaccines and intercurrent infections, such as with herpes simplex virus, produce transient increases in HIV RNA [12, 21, 27, 29, 69]. Both the mechanism and the clinical significance of these transient bursts of viral replication have yet to be determined; however, the activation of CD4 lymphocytes to render them permissive host cells for HIV replication most likely explains these transient bursts of viral replication have yet to be determined; however, the activation of CD4 lymphocytes to render them permissive host cells for HIV replication most likely explains these transient increases in plasma HIV RNA.

The concentration of HIV RNA in the plasma remains constant because production and clearance of virus are in a steady state. Productively infected cells have a life span limited by direct effects of HIV replication or immunologic clearance. During steady state, newly infected cells balance the loss of productively infected cells in a dynamic equilibrium. The rate of production of virus is proportional to the number of productively infected cells and the virus yield per infected cell, and this virus production, in the face of constant clearance rate, thus determines the steady rate levels of virus in each infected individual [9].

Antiretroviral drugs disrupt this dynamic equilibrium. The turnover rate of circulating virus is so high that 24 h after drug initiation plasma HIV RNA levels decline exponentially [26, 54] (Fig. 2). The 24-h delay is due in part to the time it takes for drug to be absorbed and reach its target, as well as the continued production of virus from cells already containing HIV reverse transcripts. Estimates of virus half-life can be made by determining rates of decline and assuming that viral replication has been completely arrested.

The early estimates of virus half-life were in the range of 1.9–2.2 days and were remarkably consistent among patients and were independent of the antiretroviral agent they had received [26, 31, 74]. In addition, viral clearance rates appeared to be independent of the level of plasma HIV RNA or CD4 T lymphocyte counts. By more frequent sampling in patients administered the protease inhibitor ritonavir, Perelson et al. [54] have further refined estimates of viral turnover. Productively infected cells are cleared with an average half-life of 1.6 days. The half-life of plasma virions is 6 h. Approximately 7×10^{10} new virions are produced each day. Thus, the apparently stable levels of HIV RNA in the plasma reflect an extraordinarily dynamic equilibrium. Because the clearance rates of virions and infected cells are similar among patients independent of immune status and disease stage, the primary determinant of the steady-state levels is the number of newly infected cells and their virus yields generated each day. The factors that account for the differences among individuals have not been identified.

Approximately 99% of the plasma virions are produced as a result of newly infected cells turning over at a very high rate. Other cells may contribute to the remaining small proportion of virus circulating in the plasma, including latently infected cells and chronically producing cells such as macrophages. When a protease inhibitor is administered, the initial 2-week exponential decay phase is followed by a slower second phase of decay [23, 42]. The half-life of this population of cells is in the range of 2 weeks (Perelson, personal communication). A third decay phase not yet documented, could conceivably follow representing a reservoir of infected cells with even a slower turnover. Successful antiretroviral therapy is dependent on achieving sustained viral suppression in each of the cell reservoirs.

Few studies have correlated changes in circulating virus, which occur as a result of antiretroviral therapy to changes in viral burden in lymphatic tissue. In one study, concordance between lymph node and plasma levels were noted after the initiation of therapy in a small number of patients, but the limited potency of the therapy and frequency of measurements limited the ability to compare changes in these two

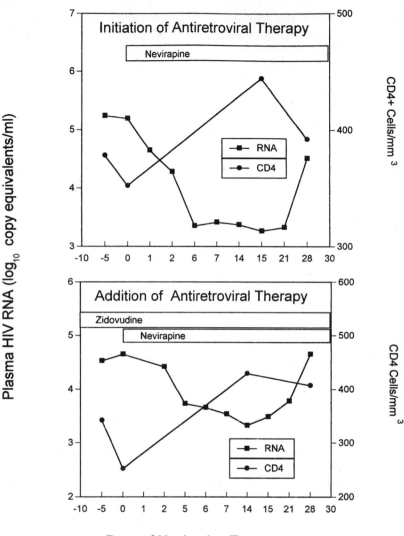

Fig. 2. The initiation of antiretroviral therapy with nevirapine (*top*) or the combination therapy with nevi-rapine and zidovudine (*bottom*). These changes in therapy produce a rapid decline of levels in HIV RNA because of disruption of the dynamic equilibrium of HIV production and clearance. Evidence for antiviral activity of new compounds cam be determined within 2 weeks, and the effect of therapy on viral burden can be rapidly assessed in patient management. Selection of virus resistant to nevirapine produces diminished virus suppression by 4 weeks, showing the rapid shifts in virus populations that can emerge under selective drug pressure. (Figure reproduced with permission from the American College of Physicians [25])

compartments [10]. The number of circulating virions is proportional to the production of virus (assuming clearance is constant); therefore, viral burden in the lymphatics, the presumed source of new infection, should be proportional to circulating virus. Changes paralleling those observed in the plasma after initiation of therapy would expected to be present in the lymph nodes assuming that the clearance between these compartments is similar. This hypothesis is currently being tested in clinical trials of potent combination antiretroviral regimens.

Resistance

With 10^{10} virions produced daily and an estimated mutation rate of 10^{-4}–10^{-5} per nucleoside per replication cycle, Coffin [9] has estimated that every possible single point mutation occurs between 10^4 and 10^5 times per day in an HIV-infected patient. Each of these genetic variants is less fit than the wild-type virus; otherwise it would be the predominant population. The relative fitness of a genetic variant changes drastically with the imposition of a selective pressure such as drug therapy, allowing a minority population to rapidly emerge. Coffin has further argued that the evolution of an HIV population is less dependent on the high mutation rate than upon the magnitude of replication of a genetically complex population in the presence of selective pressures.

Entirely consistent with these predictions were observations made when patients were administered the non-nucleoside reverse transcriptase inhibitor nevirapine, a drug known to lose 100-fold activity in vitro against HIV with a nucleotide substitution at codon 181 of the reverse transcriptase gene [61]. After nevirapine administration, there was an exponential decline in HIV RNA with a nadir of a two-log reduction in HIV RNA levels from baseline at 2 weeks. HIV RNA levels then began to rise as early as 14 days after treatment. Initially, complex mixtures of virus containing nevirapine-resistant mutants emerged, but then a more homogenous nevirapine-resistant population with a tyrosine to cysteine substitution was established [7, 62]. In patients receiving nevirapine monotherapy, the Y181C appeared to be the most fit population. In contrast, when zidovudine and nevirapine are administered concomitantly, viral populations with mutations at positions other than 181 emerged. Because the 181 mutation appears to increase susceptibility to zidovudine of zidovudine-resistant virus, mutants resistant to nevirapine at non-181 codons are more fit in the face of combination therapy with nevirapine plus zidovudine.

Lamivudine (3TC) also rapidly selects for resistance when viral suppression is incomplete. Within 5–7 days of drug administration a mutant population with M184I substitution emerges [66, 72]. This mutant is quickly replaced by more fit M184V mutant and HIV RNA levels increase back to pretreatment levels. When lamivudine is administered in conjunction with zidovudine, viral suppression is maintained despite the appearance of the M184V mutant. The explanation for these observations have not been fully elucidated but may include suppression of zidovudine resistance due to mutational interactions [40].

In contrast to lamivudine, nevirapine and other nonnucleoside analogues where single point mutations are capable of conferring drug resistance, multiple mutations are necessary to confer high-level resistance to zidovudine and the protease inhibitors [11, 38, 39]. Pre-existing drug-resistant mutants to most antiretroviral agents have been identified in small proportions of untreated patients [48, 49]. Presumably multiple drug-resistant mutants occur at a lower frequency than in single drug-resistant mutants. Recombination could accelerate the rate of acquisition of high-level resistance to multiple drugs [45]. Resistance to the drugs like zidovudine where multiple mutations are necessary typically evolves over a period of months as compared to years. The frequency of zidovudine resistance is dependent on disease stage and CD4 cell count

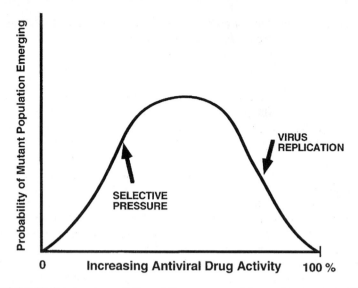

Fig. 3. The relationship between drug activity and the emergence of drug-resistant mutants. (Figure reproduced with permission from Elsevier Science B.V. [58])

which probably reflects the more rapid selection of mutants in patients with a higher viral burden [60].

The selection of drug-resistant mutants requires both adequate drug activity and continuing virus replication (Fig. 3). Until recently antiretroviral therapy for HIV produced 0.3 to 0.7 log reductions in plasma HIV RNA. With the availability of more potent chemotherapy, drug combinations are now able to effectively suppress HIV replication to levels in which HIV RNA is not detectable in the plasma using commercially available assays. Ongoing studies will define the level of viral replication in the lymph nodes and other potential reservoirs such as the central nervous system in these patients for whom the virus can no longer be detected in the plasma for periods of greater than 1 year. Resistant mutants may be present at low levels in these patients or alternatively the nearly complete suppression in viral replication produced by these more potent compounds may have reduced the burden of HIV to a level where selection will occur over a very long time period or not at all. If this is the case, then resistance to drugs such as lamivudine and nevirapine which normally occurs very rapidly may be prevented when they are used in combination with potent agents. Recent data from clinical trials support this hypothesis.

Implications for antiviral therapy

Drug development

The clinical development of the most recently approved antiretroviral agents was significantly influenced by the availability of quantitative assays for HIV RNA and the clearer understanding of HIV dynamics. Early phase I/II studies of antiretroviral drugs assessing the activity against HIV in early drug development relied on the measurement of HIV p24 antigen. This marker is only present in a small proportion of HIV-infected patients and levels of p24 are not predictive of disease progression. Quantitative measures of HIV RNA are now used to evaluate drugs for evidence of antiretroviral activity. The use of this assay offers many advantages: nearly all previously untreated patients have detectable HIV RNA levels; an assessment of antiretroviral activity can be made easily in a 4-week study; and the dynamic range (10^2–10^6 copies/ml) and precision of the assay allows for comparison among drugs. Thus, compounds which show no evidence of antiviral activity can be discarded early in drug development.

Fortunately for HIV-infected patients in developed countries, prophylaxis has successfully reduced the incidence of many opportunistic infections. Thus, "clinical endpoints" often used as a measure of efficacy in phase III clinical trials are less frequent and very large trials of thousands of patients are necessary in studies comparing various drug regimens. When HIV RNA is utilized as the primary measure of efficacy, smaller and more efficient studies can be conducted comparing various treatment regimens. Changes in HIV RNA levels produced by pharmacologic interventions are increasingly relied upon for regulatory approval of drugs prior to the completion of clinical endpoint studies.

What is the evidence that suppression of HIV RNA will confer clinical benefit? Multiple large trials addressing this important question using a variety of antiretroviral therapies have all come to the same conclusion. A greater reduction in HIV RNA is associated with a slower progression to HIV-related complications [13, 24, 34, 50, 75]. The AIDS Clinical Trials Group Study (ACTG) 175 compared the clinical outcome and survival of 2,467 HIV-infected patients with 200–500 CD4 cells/mm^3 randomly assigned to one of four nucleoside regimens [24, 34]. In a subset of these patients frequent assessments of HIV RNA were made throughout the course of the study. There was an 80% reduction in the relative risk of HIV disease progression in those patients who had at least a one log treatment-related reduction in HIV RNA. In another study which retrospectively evaluated HIV RNA as a predictor of disease progression in patients randomized to immediate versus deferred zidovudine therapy every 0.5 log reduction in HIV RNA was associated with a 63% reduction in the relative hazard of clinical disease progression [50]. In these and other studies changes in HIV RNA were more powerful and independent predictors of disease progression than CD4 cell counts. These results support the regulatory approval of compounds based on HIV RNA measurements. It is important to note, however, that other factors independent of HIV RNA levels are predictors of disease progression, such as syncytium phenotype and zidovudine susceptibility [16, 59].

Therapeutic strategies

Most would agree that achieving prolonged suppression of HIV and delay of HIV-related complications is the cornerstone of successful antiretroviral therapy. Exactly how to accomplish this goal is an area of active discussion and substantial controversy. As few as 2 years ago, there was great controversy surrounding the use of any antiretroviral therapy in asymptomatic patients. This debate was in part fueled by the low potency of zidovudine monotherapy which suppresses viral replication by 0.5 log for periods of less than a year [22, 59]. The arguments against the use of early antiretroviral therapy are no longer valid because of the availability of multiple potent antiretroviral agents which can be used in combination to achieve viral suppression for prolonged periods. Furthermore, these agents may restore some level of immunocompetence, halt HIV disease progression, and reduce mortality in advanced patients.

Maximal viral suppression requires combinations of the currently available antiretroviral agents. Interruptions of therapy when virus is incompletely suppressed leads to rapid increases in HIV RNA and enhances the probability that drug-resistant mutants will emerge. Combination therapy offers the advantages of a greater reduction in viral burden, and a greater chance of preventing the emergence of drug-resistant mutants when compared to monotherapy. While one nucleoside analogue such as didanosine may be nearly comparable in reducing viral burden by two- to threefold compared on two nucleosides such as zidovudine and zalcitabine, the addition of a third potent agent has now been shown in a number of trials to halt viral replication to levels that are not detectable in the plasma. For example, the triple drug combination of indinavir, zidovudine, and lamivudine is producing reductions in HIV RNA below the limits of detection of the assay (500 copies/ml) for greater than 44 weeks [23].

The durability of viral suppression is to a large part dependent on the ability of a drug regimen to prevent or suppress drug-resistant mutants. Resistance to drugs like nevirapine and lamivudine can be delayed for periods of 6 months or more when they are administered with agents that effectively and rapidly "shut down" viral replication. As monotherapy, resistance to these drugs predictably develops within a week of the administration of monotherapy. Therefore, to prevent the emergence of resistance and protect the potent antiretroviral activity of these drugs, they are optimally utilized with at least two other drugs to which the patient has not been exposed. In some cases, a single potent drug such as ritonavir or indinavir could potentially be useful in this regard. Based on the dynamics, administering a combination of all drugs at one time is highly preferable because delaying one drug by as little as a few days could permit outgrowth of a mutant population. Directly supervised therapy may need to be implemented, particularly early in the course of treatment with these aggressive regimens where compliance is critical. This approach has been highly successful in preventing the emergence of multidrug-resistant *Mycobacterium tuberculosis* and may be effective in achieving the same goal in the treatment of HIV.

The availability of at least nine antiretroviral agents now raises the possibility of entirely new therapeutic strategies. At present, antiretroviral agents are being used sequentially and changes are guided by the development of clinical symptoms, declining CD4 cell counts, and increases in HIV RNA. The sequential use of drugs provides a greater opportunity for the selection of increasingly resistant virus. A preferable approach may be to use an intensive drug combination initially to inhibit viral replication rapidly and effectively and to prevent the emergence of drug-resistant mutants (Fig. 4). This is analogous to the induction phase of antituberculous therapy or chemotherapy for malignancies. Once viral replication has been reduced to low levels a less-intensive maintenance regimen may be sufficient to sustain viral suppression for prolonged periods and conceivably to eradicate HIV altogether. The feasibility of either maintenance therapy or curative treatment will require systematic investigation. Patients who fail in this attempt to obtain complete suppression then would be "reinduced" with another combination regimen which would have predictable activity against drug-resistant mutants. The dynamics of virus turnover in reservoirs (i.e., macrophages and lymph tissue) of HIV are likely to be important determinants of the ability of a maintenance regimen to successfully sustain viral suppression in this setting. Once HIV RNA is no longer detectable in the plasma, the duration of ther-

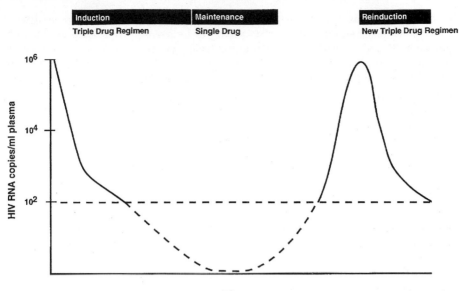

Induction	Maintenance	Reinduction
Triple Drug Regimen	Single Drug	New Triple Drug Regimen

Fig. 4. Schematic of strategy of antiretroviral therapeutic designed to maximize viral suppression and reduce long-term exposure to multiple drugs. Therapy is initiated with a triple drug regimen which suppresses virus to a level undetectable in the plasma. A rapid decline in HIV RNA is followed by a slower decay phase reflecting the effect of drugs on infected cells with difference half lives. After a period of "induction," "maintenance" therapy may be adequate to sustain viral suppression and prevent the outgrowth of resistant mutants. If therapy is withdrawn or maintenance therapy only partially suppresses virus, "escape" mutants will readily emerge requiring re-induction. Determining HIV activity in lymph node aspirates or biopsy samples may be critical in determining the optimal timeline of such a therapeutic strategy. This schematic does not reflect current practice but will be evaluated in clinical trials

apy necessary to halt viral replication in the lymph nodes is not known. Moreover, eradication will require successful suppression of viral replication in pharmacologic sanctuaries such as the central nervous system. Only a year or two ago, it was inconceivable that therapies would be available to experimentally address these important issues. Clinical trials are now ongoing to answer these questions which are pivotal to designing future therapeutic strategies.

Implications for clinical management

A single measurement of HIV RNA and CD4 cell count provides important prognostic information; sequential measures can be used to assist the management of HIV disease [64]. Prior guidelines regarding when to initiate antiretroviral therapy were based on CD4 cell count determinations. Using these recommendations, antiretroviral therapy is uniformly withheld in HIV-infected patients with greater than 500 CD4 cells/mm^3. New information has forced revision of these guidelines [6].

The entire rationale for withholding therapy in HIV-infected patients is brought into question with our new insights into HIV dynamics. Low levels of HIV RNA on the whole predict a slow progression of disease; however, there is variability even among identical HIV RNA levels for any one individual in the course of disease. Certain virus phenotypes (i.e., syncytium inducing) are associated with more rapid disease progressions, but the remainder of the variability in disease progression remains unexplained. If new methods could definitively identify infected patients unlikely to progress, the rationale for withholding therapy would be stronger. With the availability of drug combinations that effectively suppress virus replication, delay resistance, and potentially preserve immunologic function, deferring therapy may become less attractive. The arguments for initiating therapy early extend to primary infection where virus suppression can be achieved and could result in the greatest preservation of immunologic function [55]. Even in patients with primary infection and early asymptomatic HIV disease who received zidovudine, a weak agent as monotherapy compared to available combination regimens, HIV disease progression was delayed compared to placebo [14, 35].

The HIV RNA is also a potentially powerful tool for clinicians managing HIV-infected patients. The optimal frequency of monitoring requires an understanding of HIV dynamics. Without therapeutic intervention of immune activation HIV RNA levels remain relatively stable over a period of months; the biologic variability is within 0.3 log. When effective antiretroviral therapy is initiated HIV RNA levels drop within 48 h. For monotherapy with the current available nonprotease inhibitors, peak reductions in HIV RNA are observed at approximately 2 weeks. By 4–8 weeks, levels increase to steady-state levels below pre-treatment HIV RNA. With protease inhibitors and combination regimens which prevent the emergence of escape mutant virus, a slower decline in HIV RNA continues over a period of months (see above). In one study of patients with CD4 cells of $50–400/mm^3$ and a mean baseline HIV RNA of 10^4 copies/ml plasma, HIV RNA levels become undetectable in 5–6 months in patients receiving a triple drug therapy combination [4]. Thus, in untreated patients where the goal is to achieve complete viral suppression in the plasma, post-treatment levels of HIV RNA should be obtained after 5–6 months of therapy. In patients treated with prior antiretroviral therapy, where antiviral response is less certain, a qualitative assessment of any treatment response with a new regimen can be made at 2 weeks. The optimal frequency of monitoring in patients with undetectable virus or on regimens where virus suppression is incomplete awaits more definitive clinical trial data, but every 3–4 months has been recommended [64].

Decreases in plasma HIV RNA levels are associated with proportional increases in CD4 cell counts. With nucleoside therapy, peak CD4 cell count increases occur at about 4–8 weeks and lag behind HIV RNA reductions which occur at 2 weeks [22]. The more potent triple-drug antiretroviral regimens which suppress viral replication to undetectable plasma levels result in CD4 cell count increases in the 100–200 range. Parallel to the dynamics of HIV RNA in the plasma, increases in CD4 cell count are initially rapid but then begin to increase more slowly over time. Whether the functional capacity of these cells are intact and provide complete protection against opportunistic infections is unknown at present.

Effective viral suppression may permit only partial reconstitution of immunologic function which may be more dependent on prior immunologic destruction. Furthermore, improvements in immunologic function may extend years beyond clearance of detectable plasma HIV RNA. A thorough understanding of HIV RNA dynamics, a familiarity with a large number of antiretroviral agents, and a clearer picture of the dynamics and extent of immune restoration with suppressive chemotherapy of HIV replication will be critical to the skillful management of HIV- infected patients in the future.

Conclusions

Recent insights into HIV dynamics have been facilitated by the HIV RNA quantitative assay, have revised models pathogenesis, revolutionized drug development, and have been applied directly in the clinical setting. The prospect of shifting patients from a prognosis of a progressive fatal infection to indefinite non- progression as well as understanding of the pathogenetic basis of these dramatic changes indicates remarkable progress in just a few years.

Acknowledgements. The authors thank Janice Menendez for manuscript preparation and Darcia Smith for technical assistance. This work was supported by grants AI 27670, AI 36214, AI 29164 (Center for AIDS Research), and AI 30457 from the National Institutes of Health, by the Research Center for AIDS and HIV Infection for the San Diego Veterans Affairs Medical Center; and by the California Universitywide Taskforce on AIDS.

References

1. Armstrong JA, Horne R (1984) Follicular dendritic cells and virus-like particles in AIDS-related lymphadenopathy. Lancet II:370
2. Bagasra O, Hauptman SP, Lischner HW, Sachs M, Pomerantz RJ (1992) Detection of human immunodeficiency virus type 1 provirus in mononuclear cells by in situ polymerase chain reaction. N Engl J Med 326:1385
3. Baroni CD, Pezzella F, Mirolo M, Ruco LP, Rossi GB (1986) Immunohistochemical demonstration of p24 HTLV III major core protein in different cell types within lymph nodes from patients with lymphadenopathy syndrome (LAS). Histopathology 10:5
4. Biberfeld P, Chayt KJ, Marselle LM, Biberfeld G, Gallo RC, Harper ME (1986) HTLV-III expression in infected lymph nodes and relevance to pathogenesis of lymphadenopathy. Am J Pathol 125:436
5. Cao Y, Qin L, Zhang L, Safrit J, Ho DD (1995) Virologic and immunologic characterization of long-term survivors of human immunodeficiency virus type 1 infection. N Engl J Med 332:201
6. Carpenter CCJ, Fischl MA, Hammer SM, Hirsch MS, Jacobsen DM, Katzenstein DA, Montaner J, Richman DD, Saag MS, Schooley RT, Thompson MA, Vella S, Yeni PG, Volberding PA, for the International AIDS Society - USA (1996) Antiretroviral therapy for HIV infection in 1996. JAMA 275:(in press)
7. Cheeseman SH, Havlir DV, McLaughlin M, Greenough TC, Sullivan JL, Hall D, Hattox SE, Spector SA, Stein DS, Myers M, Richman DD (1995) Phase I/II evaluation of nevirapine alone and in combination with zidovudine for infection with human immunodeficiency virus. J Acquir Immune Defic Syndr Hum Retrovirol 8:141
8. Clark SJ, Saag MS, Decker WD, Campbell-Hill S, Roberson JL, Veldkamp PJ, Kappes JC, Hahn BH, Shaw GM (1991) High titers of cytopathic virus in plasma of patients with symptomatic primary HIV
9. Coffin JM (1995) HIV population dynamics in vivo: implications for genetic variation, pathogenesis, and therapy. Science 267:483
10. Cohen OJ, Pantaleo G, Holodniy M, Schnittman S, Niu M, Graziosi C, Pavlakis GN, Lalezari J, Bartlett JA, Steigbigel RT (1995) Decreased human immunodeficiency virus type 1 plasma viremia during antiretroviral therapy reflects downregulation of viral replication in lymphoid tissue. Proc Natl Acad Sci USA 92:6017
11. Condra JH, Schleif WA, Blahy OM, Gabryelski LJ, Graham DJ, Quintero JC, Rhodes A, Robbins HL, Roth E, Shivaprakash M (1995) In vivo emergence of HIV-1 variants resistant to multiple protease inhibitors. Nature 374:569
12. Coombs RW, Collier AC, Allain JP, Nikora B, Leuther M, Gjerset GF, Corey L (1989) Plasma viremia in human immunodeficiency virus infection. N Engl J Med 321:1626
13. Coombs RW, Welles SL, Hooper C, et al (1996) Association of plasma human immunodeficiency virus type-1 RNA level with risk of clinical progression in patients with advanced infection. J Infect Dis: in press

14. Cooper DA, Gatell JM, Kroon S, Clumeck N, Millard J, Goebel FD, Bruun JN, Stingl G, Melville RL, Gonzalez-Lahoz J, Stevens JW, Fiddian AP (1993) Zidovudine in persons with asymptomatic HIV infection and CD4$^+$ cell counts greater than 400 cubic millimeter. N Engl J Med 329:297
15. Daar ES, Moudgil T, Meyer RD, Ho DD (1991) Transient high levels of viremia in patients with primary human immunodeficiency virus type 1 infection. N Engl J Med 324:961
16. D'Aquila RT, Johnson VA, Welles SL, Japour AJ, Kuritzkes DR, DeGruttola V, Reichelderfer PS, Coombs RW, Crumpacker CS, Kahn JO (1995) Zidovudine resistance and HIV-1 disease progression during antiretroviral therapy. AIDS Clinical Trials Group Protocol 116B/117 Team and the Virology Committee Resistance Working Group. Ann Intern Med 122:401
17. Delwart EL, Sheppard HW, Walker BD, Goudsmit J, Mullins JI (1994) Human immunodeficiency virus type 1 evolution in vivo tracked by DNA heteroduplex mobility assays. J Virol 68:6672
18. Demarest JF, Daucher M, Vaccarezza M, Graziosi C, Cohen OJ, Tambussi G, Corey L, Pantaleo G, Fauci AS (1996) Qualitative differences in the primary immune response to HIV infection may be predictive of subsequent clinical outcome. Abstracts of the 3rd Conference on Retroviruses and Opportunistic Infections, Washington, DC, Jan 29–Feb 1. IDSA Alexandria, VA, abstr. no. 420
19. Dewar RL, Highbarger HC, Sarmiento MD, Todd JA, Vasudevachari MB, Davey RTJ, Kovacs JA, Salzman NP, Lane HC, Urdea MS (1994) Application of branched DNA signal amplification to monitor human immunodeficiency virus type 1 burden in human plasma. J Infect Dis 170:1172
20. Di Stefano M, Norkrans G, Chiodi F, Hagberg L, Nielsen C, Svennerholm B (1993) Zidovudine-resistant variants of HIV-1 in brain [letter]. Lancet 342:865
21. Embretson J, Zupancic M, Ribas JL, Burke A, Racz P, Tenner-Tacz K, Haase AT (1993) Massive covert infection of helper T lymphocytes and macrophages by HIV during the incubation period of AIDS. Nature 362:359
22. Eron JJ, Benoit SL, Jemsek J, MacArthur RD, Santana J, Quinn JB, Kuritzkes DR, Fallon MA, Rubin M (1995) Treatment with lamivudine, zidovudine, or both in HIV-positive patients with 200 to 500 CD4$^+$ cell per cubic millimeter. North American Working Party. N Engl J Med 333:1662
23. Gulick R, Mellors J, Havlir D, Eron J, Gonzalez C, McMahon D, Richman D, Valentine F, Jonas L, Meibohm A, Chiou R, Deutsch P, Emini E, Chodakewitz J (1996) Potent and sustained antiretroviral activity of indinavir (IDV) in combination with zidovudine (ZDV) and lamivudine (3TC). Abstracts of the 3rd Conference on Retroviruses and Opportunistic Infections, Washington, DC, Jan 29–Feb 1. IDSA Alexandria, VA, LB7
24. Hammer S, Katzenstein D, Hughes M, Gundacker H, Hirsch M, Merigan T (1995) Nucleoside monotherapy versus combination therapy in HIV-infected adults: a randomized, double-blind, placebo-controlled trial in persons with CD4 cell counts 200–500/mm^3. Abstracts of the 35th Interscience Conference on Antimicrobial Agents and Chemotherapy, San Francisco, Calif., Sept 17–20. ASM Washington, DC, no. LB-1
25. Havlir DV, Richman DD (1996) Viral dynamics of HIV: implications for drug development and therapeutic strategies. Ann Intern Med 124:984
26. Havlir D, Eastman S, Richman DD (1995) HIV-1 kinetics: rates of production and clearance of viral populations in asymptomatic patients treated with nevirapine. Abstracts of the 2nd National Conference on Human Retroviruses and Related Infections, Washington, DC, Jan 29–Feb 2. ASM Washington, DC, abstr. no. 229
27. Henrard DR, Daar E, Farzadegan H, Clark SJ, Phillips J, Shaw GM, Busch MP (1995) Virologic and immunologic characterization of symptomatic and asymptomatic primary HIV-1 infection. J Acquir Immune Defic Syndr Hum Retrovirol 9:305
28. Henrard DR, Phillips JF, Muenz LR, Blattner WA, Wiesner D, Eyster ME, Goedert JJ (1995) Natural history of HIV-1 cell-free viremia. JAMA 274:554
29. Ho DD (1992) HIV-1 viraemia and influenza [letter]. Lancet 339:1549
30. Ho DD, Moudgil T, Alam M (1989) Quantitation of human immunodeficiency virus type 1 in the blood of infected persons. N Engl J Med 321:1621
31. Ho DD, Neumann AU, Perelson AS, Chen W, Leonard JM, Markowitz M (1995) Rapid turnover of plasma virions and CD4 lymphocytes in HIV-1 infection. Nature 373:123
32. Hollander H, Levy JA (1987) Neurologic abnormalities and recovery of human immunodeficiency virus from cerebrospinal fluid. Ann Intern Med 106:692
33. Jurriaans S, Van Gemen B, Weverling GJ, Van Strijp D, Nara P, Coutinho R, Koot M, Schuitemaker H, Goudsmit J (1994) The natural history of HIV-1 infection: virus load and virus phenotype independent determinants of clinical course? Virology 204:223

34. Katzenstein D, Hammer S, Hughes M, Gundacker H, Jackson B, Merigan T, Hirsch M, for the ACTG 175 Virology Team (1995) Plasma virion RNA in response to early antiretroviral drug therapy in ACTG 175. Do changes in virus load parallel clinical and immunologic outcomes? Abstracts of the 35th Interscience Conference on Antimicrobial Agents and Chemotherapy, San Francisco, Calif., Sept 17–20. ASM Washington, DC, abstr. no. LB-2
35. Kinloch-De Loes S, Hirschel BJ, Hoen B, Cooper DA, Tindall B, Carr A, Saurat JH, Clumeck N, Lazzarin A, Mathiesen L (1995) A controlled trial of zidovudine in primary human immunodeficiency virus infection. N Engl J Med 333:408
36. Kirchhoff F, Greenough TC, Brettler DB, Sullivan JL, Desrosiers RC (1995) Brief report: absence of intact *nef* sequences in a long-term survivor with nonprogressive HIV-1 infection. N Engl J Med 332:228
37. Koup RA, Safrit JT, Cao Y, Andrews CA, McLeod G, Borkowsky W, Farthing C, Ho DD (1994) Temporal association of cellular immune responses with the initial control of viremia in primary human immunodeficiency virus type 1 syndrome. J Virol 68:4650
38. Larder BA, Kemp SD (1989) Multiple mutations in HIV-1 reverse transcriptase confer high-level resistance to zidovudine (AZT). Science 246:1155
39. Larder BA, Darby G, Richman DD (1989) HIV with reduced sensitivity to zidovudine (AZT) isolated during prolonged therapy. Science 243:1731
40. Larder BA, Kemp SD, Harrigan PR (1995) Potential mechanism for sustained antiretroviral efficacy of AZT-3TC combination therapy. Science 269:696
41. Le Tourneau A, Audouin J, Diebold J, Marche C, Tricottet V, Reynes M (1986) LAV-like viral particles in lymph node germinal centers in patients with the persistent lymphadenopathy syndrome and the acquired immunodeficiency syndrome-related complex: an ultrastructural study of 30 cases. Hum Pathol 17:1047
42. Markowitz M, Saag M, Powderly WG, Hurley AM, Hsu A, Valdes JM, Henry D, Sattler F, La Marca A, Leonard JM (1995) A preliminary study of ritonavir, an inhibitor of HIV-1 protease, to treat HIV-1 infection. N Engl J Med 333:1534
43. Mellors JW, Kingsley LA, Rinaldo CRJ, Todd JA, Hoo BS, Kokka RP, Gupta P (1995) Quantitation of HIV-1 RNA in plasma predicts outcome after seroconversion. Ann Intern Med 122:573
44. Mellors JW, Rinaldo Jr. CR, Gupta P, White RM, Todd JA, Kingsley LA (1996) Prognosis in HIV-1 infection predicted by the quantity of virus in plasma. Science 272:1167
45. Moutouh L, Corbeil J, Richman DD (1996) Recombination leads to the rapid emergence of HIV-1 dually resistant mutants under selective drug pressure. Proc Natl Acad Sci USA 93:6106
46. Mulder J, McKinney N, Christopherson C, Sninsky J, Greenfield L, Kwok S (1994) Rapid and simple PCR assay for quantitation of human immunodeficiency virus type 1 RNA in plasma: application to acute retroviral infection. J Clin Microbiol 32:292
47. Munoz A, Kirby AJ, He YD, Margolick JB, Visscher BR, Rinaldo CR, Kaslow RA, Phair JP (1995) Long-term survivors with HIV-1 infection: incubation period and longitudinal patterns of CD4+ lymphocytes. J Acquir Immune Defic Syndr Hum Retrovirol 8:496
48. Najera I, Richman DD, Olivares I, Rojas JM, Peinado MA, Perucho M, Najera R, Lopez-Galindez C (1994) Natural occurrence of drug-resistant mutations in the reverse transcriptase of human immunodeficiency virus type 1 isolates. AIDS Res Hum Retroviruses 10:1479
49. Najera I, Holguin A, Quinones-Mateu ME, Munoz-Fernandez MA, Najera R, Lopez-Galindez C, Domingo E (1995) *pol* gene quasispecies of human immunodeficiency virus: mutations associated with drug resistance in virus from patients undergoing no drug therapy. J Virol 69:23
50. O'Brien WA, Hartigan PM, Martin D, Esinhart J, Hill A, Benoit S, Rubin M, Simberkoff MS, Hamilton JD (1996) Changes in plasma HIV-1 RNA and CD4+ lymphocyte counts and the risk of progression to AIDS. Veterans Affairs Cooperative Study Group on AIDS. N Engl J Med 334:426
51. Pantaleo G, Graziosi C, Demarest JF, Butini L, Montroni M, Fox CH, Orenstein JM, Kotler DP, Fauci AS (1993) HIV infection is active and progressive in lymphoid tissue during the clinically latent stage of disease. Nature 362:355
52. Pantaleo G, Menzo S, Vaccarezza M, Graziosi C, Cohen OJ, Demarest JF, Montefiori D, Orenstein JM, Fox C, Schrager LK (1995) Studies in subjects with long-term nonprogressive human immunodeficiency virus infection. N Engl J Med 332:209
53. Patterson BK, Till M, Otto P, Goolsby C, Furtado MR, McBride LJ, Wolinsky SM (1993) Detection of HIV-1 DNA and messenger RNA in individual cells by PCR-driven in situ hybridization and flow cytometry. Science 260:976

54. Perelson AS, Neumann AU, Markowitz M, Leonard JM, Ho DD (1996) HIV-1 dynamics in vivo: virion clearance rate, infected cell lifetime, and viral generation time. Science 271:1582
55. Perrin L, Rakik A, Yerly S, Baumberger C, Loes SK, Pechere M, Hirschel B (1996) Combined therapy with zidovudine and L-697,661 in primary HIV infection. AIDS:(in press)
56. Phillips AN (1996) Reduction of HIV concentration during acute infection: independence from a specific immune response. Science 271:497
57. Richman DD (1995) Drug resistance in relation to pathogenesis. AIDS [Suppl A]:S49
58. Richman DD (1996) The implications of drug resistance for strategies of combination antiviral chemotherapy. Antiviral Res 29:31
59. Richman DD, Bozzette SA (1994) The impact of the syncytium-inducing phenotype of human immunodeficiency virus on disease progression. J Infect Dis 169:968
60. Richman DD, Grimes JM, Lagakos SW (1990) Effect of stage of disease and drug dose on zidovudine susceptibilities of isolates of human immunodeficiency virus. J Acquir Immune Defic Syndr Hum Retrovirol 3:743
61. Richman D, Shih CK, Lowy I, Rose J, Prodanovich P, Goff S, Griffin J (1991) Human immunodeficiency virus type 1 mutants resistant to nonnucleoside inhibitors of reverse transcriptase arise in tissue culture. Proc Natl Acad Sci USA 88:11241
62. Richman DD, Havlir D, Corbeil J, Looney D, Ignacio C, Spector SA, Sullivan J, Cheeseman S, Barringer K, Pauletti D, Shih CK, Myers M, Griffin J (1994) Nevirapine resistance mutations of human immunodeficiency virus type 1 selected during therapy. J Virol 68:1660
63. Saag MS, Crain MJ, Decker WD, Campbell-Hill S, Robinson S, Brown WE, Leuther M, Whitley RJ, Hahn BH, Shaw GM (1991) High-level viremia in adults and children infected with human immunodeficiency virus: relation to disease stage and CD4$^+$ lymphocyte levels. J Infect Dis 164:72
64. Saag MS, Holodniy M, Kuritzkes DR, O'Brien WA, Coombs R, Poscher ME, Jacobsen DM, Shaw GM, Richman DD, Volberding PA (1996) HIV viral load markers in clinical practice. Nature Med 2:625
65. Schacker TW, Hughes J, Shea T, Corey L (1996) Virologic course of primary HIV infection. Abstracts of the 3rd Conference on Retroviruses and Opportunistic Infections, Washington, DC, Jan 29–Feb 1. IDSA Alexandria, VA, abstr. no. 480
66. Schuurman R, Nijhuis M, van Leeuwen R, Schipper P, de Jong D, Collis P, Danner SA, Mulder J, Loveday C, Christopherson C (1995) Rapid changes in human immunodeficiency virus type 1 RNA load and appearance of drug-resistant virus populations in persons treated with lamivudine (3TC). J Infect Dis 171:1411
67. Sei S, Kleiner DE, Kopp JB, Chandra R, Klotman PE, Yarchoan R, Pizzo PA, Mitsuya H (1994) Quantitative analysis of viral burden in tissues from adults and children with symptomatic human immunodeficiency virus type 1 infection assessed by polymerase chain reaction. J Infect Dis 170:325
68. Sonnerborg AB, Ehrnst AC, Bergdahl SK, Pehrson PO, Skoldenberg BR, Strannegard OO (1988) HIV isolation from cerebrospinal fluid in relation to immunological deficiency and neurological symptoms. AIDS 2:89
69. Stanley SK, Ostrowski MA, Justement JS, Gantt K, Hedayati S, Mannix M, Roche K, Schwartzentruber DJ, Fox CH, Fauci AS (1996) Effect of immunization with a common recall antigen on viral expression in patients infected with human immunodeficiency virus type 1. N Engl J Med 334:1222
70. Tenner-Racz K, Racz P, Dietrich M, Kern P (1985) Altered follicular dendritic cells and virus-like particles in AIDS and AIDS-related lymphadenopathy [letter]. Lancet 1:105
71. Tenner-Racz K, Racz P, Bofill M, Schulz-Meyer A, Dietrich M, Kern P, Weber J, Pinching AJ, Veronese-Dimarzo F, Popovic M (1986) HTLV-III/LAV viral antigens in lymph nodes of homosexual men with persistent generalized lymphadenopathy and AIDS. Am J Pathol 123:9
72. Tisdale M, Kemp SD, Parry NR, Larder BA (1993) Rapid in vitro selection of human immunodeficiency virus type 1 resistant to 3'-thiacytidine inhibitors due to a mutation in the YMDD region of reverse transcriptase. Proc Natl Acad Sci USA 90:5653
73. Van Gemen B, Van Beuningen R, Nabbe A, Van Strijp D, Jurriaans S, Lens P, Kievits T (1994) A one-tube quantitative HIV-1 RNA NASBA nucleic acid amplification assay using electrochemi luminescent (ECL) labelled probes. J Virol Methods 49:157
74. Wei X, Ghosh SK, Taylor ME, Johnson VA, Emini EA, Deutsch P, Lifson JD, Bonhoeffer S, Nowak MA, Hahn BH, Saag MS, Shaw GM (1995) Viral dynamics in human immunodeficiency virus type 1 infection. Nature 373:117

75. Welles SL, Jackson JB, Yen-Lieberman B (1996) Prognostic value of plasma HIV-1 RNA levels in patients with advanced HIV-1 disease and with little or no zidovudine therapy. J Infect Dis:(in press)
76. Wildemann B, Haas J, Ehrhart K, Wagner H, Lynen N, Storch-Hagenlocher B (1993) In vivo comparison of zidovudine resistance mutations in blood and CSF of HIV-1 infected patients. Neurology 43:2659
77. Wiley CA, Schrier RD, Nelson JA, Lampert PW, Oldstone MB (1986) Cellular localization of human immunodeficiency virus infection within the brains of acquired immune deficiency syndrome patients. Proc Natl Acad Sci USA 83:7089
78. Winters MA, Tan LB, Katzenstein DA, Merigan TC (1993) Biological variation and quality control of plasma human immunodeficiency virus type 1 RNA quantitation by reverse transcriptase polymerase chain reaction. J Clin Microbiol 31:2960
79. Wolinsky SM, Wike CM, Korber BT, Hutto C, Parks WP, Rosenblum LL, Kunstman KJ, Furtado MR, Munoz JL (1992) Selective transmission of human immunodeficiency virus type-1 variants from mothers to infants [see comments]. Science 255:1134
80. Wolinsky SM, Korber BT, Neumann AU, Daniels M, Kunstman KJ, Whetsell AJ, Furtado MR, Cao Y, Ho DD, Safrit JT, Koup RA (1996) Adaptive evolution of human immunodeficiency virus-type 1 during the natural course of infection. Science 272:537
81. Wong JK, Fitch NJS, Torriani F, Havlir DV, Richman DD (1994) Discordance of RT sequences conferring ZDV resistance in proviral DNA form brain and spleen. Abstracts of the 3rd International Workshop on HIV Drug Resistance, Kauai, Hawaii, Aug 2–5. abstr. no. 46
82. Zhu T, Mo H, Wang N, Nam DS, Cao Y, Koup RA, Ho DD (1993) Genotypic and phenotypic characterization of HIV-1 patients with primary infection. Science 261:1179

Immune dysregulation and CD4+ T cell loss in HIV-1 infection

Linde Meyaard[1,*], Frank Miedema[1,2]

[1]Department of Clinical Viro-Immunology, Central Laboratory of the Netherlands Red Cross Blood Transfusion Service and the Laboratory of Experimental and Clinical Immunology of the University of Amsterdam, Plesmanlaan 125, 1066 CX Amsterdam, The Netherlands
[2]Department of Human Retrovirology, Academic Medical Centre, Amsterdam, The Netherlands

Introduction

Acquired immunodeficiency syndrome (AIDS) is the clinical outcome of human immunodeficiency virus type 1 or 2 (HIV-1, HIV-2) infection. Acute infection with HIV, which may present with influenza- or mononucleosis-like symptoms [148], is followed by an asymptomatic period of a few months to more than 13 years. This asymptomatic period is characterized by declining numbers of circulating CD4+ T helper (Th) cells, eventually leading to immunodeficiency and clinical symptoms defining the AIDS diagnosis. The symptoms observed may be lymphadenopathy, infections with opportunistic pathogens, neoplasms such as Kaposi sarcoma and non-Hodgkin lymphoma, neurological symptoms and dementia. The opportunistic infections arc mainly caused by intracellular pathogens such as viruses, mycobacteria, protozoa and fungi which, as the malignancies observed, are indicative for failing cellular immunity.

T cell turnover in HIV infection

The hallmark event in AIDS pathogenesis is the loss of CD4+ cells. The risk for development of AIDS-associated symptoms increases with declining CD4+ T cell numbers [50, 105]. The very gradual loss of circulating CD4+ T cells has long been regarded as a sign that the disease process had slow dynamics with relatively little virus activity in the asymptomatic phase. New insights into virus-host interaction in HIV infection came with the novel results on viral dynamics reported by the groups of Ho and Shaw [64, 158]. They showed that treatment of relatively late stage patients with anti-viral drugs, results in rapid clearance of free virus in plasma which is accompanied by a surprisingly quick increase of the number of CD4+ T cells in

Correspondence to: F. Miedema, (address see [1] above)
* *Present address*: DNAX Research Institute, Department of Human Immunology, Palo Alto, CA 94304–1104, USA

peripheral blood even in patients with very low CD4+ T cell counts before treatment. Mathematical modelling of the kinetic data showed that turnover of plasma virions and virus-infected cells was very fast. Assuming a steady state before treatment, plasma virion half-life is now estimated to be in the order of 6 h. CD4+ T cell production was estimated to be in the order of 2×10^9 cells per day. Thus, the gradually increasing small net loss of CD4+ T cells as observed in the course of HIV infection has, since that study appeared, been interpreted to be an increasing difference between two main factors, namely the clearance and renewal of CD4+ T cells.

The interpretation of these studies, however, is hampered by our lack of quantitative information on CD4+ T cell turnover in non-infected healthy subjects. Moreover, it has been argued by others that the rapid increase in peripheral blood CD4+ T cell numbers after anti-viral treatment might be due to redistribution of cells coming from lymphoid tissues and is not due to newly formed cells derived from peripheral or thymic precursors. Preliminary results from Ho et al. [65] of phenotypic analyses of the repopulating CD4+ T cells after anti-viral therapy, in an attempt to determine where they originate from, based on the expression of activation markers or homing receptors, showed that most of the CD4+ T cells were cycling and had an activated memory phenotype which they have interpreted as evidence for post-thymic proliferation. It remains to be seen whether this interpretation is correct.

Programmed death of T cells in HIV infection

Before these studies appeared, several other observations have supported the idea of increased turnover of T cells in HIV infection through apoptosis, or programmed cell death (PCD). Ameisen and Capron [3] were the first to propose that in HIV infection interaction of soluble gp120 with CD4, previously shown to lead to impaired lymphocyte function [26], could prime CD4+ T cells for PCD, which might provide a mechanism for CD4+ T cell loss. Indeed, peripheral blood mononuclear cells (PBMC) from HIV-infected individuals die due to PCD in vitro [59, 61, 78, 94, 95, 117, 121]. PCD can be enhanced by activation in vitro with T cell receptor (TCR)/CD3 monoclonal antibodies (mAb), lectins, superantigens or ionomycin [59, 61, 94, 117]. PCD occurs in both CD4+ and CD8+ T cells and phenotypical analysis suggests that higher percentages of CD8+ cells are dying [23, 59, 94, 95].

In primary HIV infection the increased percentage of T cells dying due to apoptosis after overnight culture is high (up to 60%) and parallels transient increases of CD8+ cell numbers. Because they form the largest fraction of T cells, numerically the majority of cells dying during primary infection are activated, CD8+CD45RO+ cells. However, all CD8+ T cell subsets contain cells dying due to PCD and there is no evidence for preferential death in one specific subset of cells [78, 95]. In the asymptomatic phase of HIV infection there is a variable but, compared to HIV-negative controls, consistently increased percentage of cells dying due to PCD [59, 94, 95]. We and others have shown that PCD does not correlate with CD4+ T cell numbers in asymptomatic individuals, nor with viral load, arguing against dramatic changes in the extent of PCD with progression to disease [82, 95, 107].

Mechanisms of apoptosis of T cells in HIV infection

In HIV-infected chimpanzees, that do not develop clinical symptoms, the proportion of T cells dying due to PCD does not exceed that in non-infected animals [59, 136]. This could imply either a function for PCD in HIV pathogenesis in humans, or that PCD is a reflection of immunopathogenic events. Several hypotheses on the cause of increased PCD of T cells in human HIV infection and the contribution to AIDS pathogenesis have been proposed, including direct virus infection of cells, CD4 ligation by gp120 and excessive immune activation.

Direct viral infection. In vitro infection of T cells and T cell lines with HIV results in cell death associated with apoptosis [77, 92, 145], and pulsing of dendritic cells with HIV results in infection and apoptosis of co-cultured CD4$^+$ T cells [21]. The capacity of HIV to induce apoptosis in vitro is related to the cell line and virus strain used and is, at least in part, associated with the efficiency of virus replication in these cells [92].

Direct virus-induced cell death, however, can be excluded as the main cause of PCD of peripheral T cells in asymptomatic HIV infection. Not only is the frequency of infected cells during asymptomatic infection too low to explain the cell death observed, there seems to be no clear cut relation between elevated virus load during both acute and asymptomatic infection and increases in PCD [95]. However, in later stages of infection, with a high viral burden in T cells in lymph nodes, direct infection of cells leading to apoptosis might contribute to CD4$^+$ T cell depletion. Arguing against this is the finding that in HIV- and simian immunodeficiency virus-infected lymph nodes apoptosis occurs predominantly in bystander cells and not in the productively infected cells themselves [52]. However, HIV infection of thymocytes might lead to increased apoptotic death in the thymus, thereby affecting regeneration of the peripheral T cell compartment [16].

Apoptosis induced by viral proteins. The initial hypothesis regarding PCD in HIV infection was that interaction of soluble HIV envelope protein (gp120) with CD4 could prime T cells for PCD [3]. Mature murine lymphocytes die from PCD after stimulation via TCR/CD3 when CD4 has been previously ligated by CD4 antibodies [111]. Furthermore, addition of gp120 in vitro impairs T cell function [26, 87, 116]. Indeed in human cells, cross-linking of CD4 mAb or bound gp120 on human CD4$^+$ T cells followed by signaling through the TCR results in apoptosis in vitro [9, 117]. Expression of gp160 in a CD4$^+$ T cell line causes down-regulation of CD4 and single-cell killing due to apoptosis [81] and in vitro exposure to HIV, without infection, of a CD34$^+$ hematopoietic progenitor cell line induces apoptotic cell death [165]. In addition to the viral envelope, the virally encoded protein Tat was demonstrated to induce cell death in vitro in T cell lines and PBMC [79, 123], possibly by up-regulation of Fas expression on T cells [160].

These data all point to a role for viral proteins in inducing T cell deficiency and apoptosis. gp120-CD4 ligation might be a mechanism for apoptosis of CD4$^+$ T cells in vivo.

Immune activation. A CD4-dependent mechanism for PCD is not likely to be the only phenomenon in HIV infection. First, both CD4$^+$ and CD8$^+$ cells, with a preference for CD8$^+$ cells, are dying due to apoptosis [23, 59, 94, 107] and secondly, during primary HIV infection, the number of cells dying exceeds by far the percentage of CD4$^+$ cells present at that time [95]. CD8$^+$ T cells from HIV-infected individuals have increased expression of activation markers as CD38, HLA-DR and CD57, suggestive for continuous immune activation [128, 141]. In lymph nodes from HIV-infected individuals a relation between apoptosis and immune activation but not viral load has been reported [107]. Because the percentage of cells dying due to PCD in primary HIV infection parallels the CD8$^+$ T cell expansion, it is tempting to speculate that PCD in HIV infection reflects turn over of activated immune cells, although PCD is not confined to a specific subset expressing activation markers [78, 95].

PCD as a result of massive immune activation following acute virus infection is not specific for HIV infection since it was also demonstrated for cytomegalovirus infection in man [151] and acute lymphocytic choriomeningitis virus (LCMV) infection in mice [124], correlating with hypo- responsiveness as a result of hyperactivation of T cells in vivo. Although it was argued by Estaquier et al. [47] that CD4$^+$ cell death is specific for HIV infection, in Epstein-Barr virus (EBV) infection in humans, both CD4$^+$ and CD8$^+$ cells also die upon culture [106, 149]. Dying cells were confined to the CD45RO$^+$ population and cell death could be prevented by culture in the presence of cytokines such as interleukin (IL)-2 [12, 149]. Under these conditions, it was suggested that PCD affects the population of activated T cells that expands during the acute phase of the infection.

We propose that PCD in acute HIV infection is a reflection of immune activation leading to high turnover of cells, as is observed in acute virus infections in general. High numbers of apoptotic cells in the early stage of infection are followed by moderately increased numbers of cells dying during the asymptomatic phase, as seen in the asymptomatic phase of feline immunodeficiency virus infection in cats [13]. In asymptomatic HIV infection, PCD reflects a continuous activation leading to priming for death and deletion of responding T cells.

Turnover of activated T cells by apoptotic cell death

The mechanism by which T cells in HIV infection are driven towards apoptosis might reflect a general phenomenon of termination of the immune response upon activation. Wesselborg et al. [159] reported that while freshly isolated T cells from healthy individuals are resistant to PCD, the susceptibility of these cells for induced death increases upon activation and culture. In agreement with the observations in HIV infection, in these experiments no correlation between susceptibility for death and the expression of a specific activation marker could be demonstrated.

Several cascades of events can be envisaged by which the immune system will set stop at an initiated immune response. As suggested by findings in murine LCMV infection [124] and experimental autoimmune encephalomyelitis [40], T cell death might be a physiological response to prolonged IL-2 stimulation after massive immune activation or high antigen dose. The apoptosis-related Fas antigen is known to be preferentially expressed on previously activated or memory T cells [104]. Fas-Fas ligand (FasL) interaction might play a role by the elimination of excessive immune cells, since CD45RO$^+$ cells in acute EBV infection, known to undergo apoptosis, have increased expression of Fas [149]. In HIV-infected individuals, T cells also have an increased expression of Fas and increased percentages of cells dying in culture upon Fas ligation with anti- Fas antibodies [70].

The proto-oncogene *bcl*-2 has been identified as a controller of PCD in a variety of cell types [75]. It was proposed that the regulation of *bcl*-2 expression within the

CD45RO+ T cell population regulates cell death and survival and is a mechanism for the removal of unwanted T cells after resolution of viral disease [2]. After repeated stimulation, primed T cells lose *bcl*-2 expression, gain Fas expression and become highly susceptible for death [130], which has also recently been demonstrated for CD8+ T cells from HIV-infected individuals [15, 17]. Furthermore, a relation between low *bcl*-2 expression and enhanced cell death has been demonstrated in other viral infections [1, 142].

Importantly, we and others have observed that in HIV infection, T cells die irrespective of the expression of activation markers [78, 95]. Massive immune activation could lead to exhaustion of growth and survival factors and subsequently result in PCD. Our finding that, in vitro, growth factors could not prevent the death of cells from HIV-infected individuals, does not exclude such a mechanism but may indicate that cells from HIV-infected individuals are already irreversibly primed for PCD in vivo [95]. Other groups, however, have reported rescue of cells from HIV-infected individuals from apoptosis by combinations of growth factors [59, 61, 121]. Furthermore, apoptosis has been reported to be differentially influenced by Th1 and Th2 cytokines. Th1 cytokines and anti-Th2 cytokine antibodies were reported to inhibit programmed cell death of T cells from HIV-1-infected individuals in vitro [35, 48].

Oxidative stress has been proposed as a mediator of apoptosis [20]. Activated CD4+ and CD8+ T cells from HIV-infected individuals have glutathione deficiency [43, 140] and might be less capable of withstanding oxidative stress and, thereby, death due to PCD. Antigen-presenting cell (APC) function, regulating either proliferation and cytokine production or cell death of the responding T cell, was proposed as a mechanism to shape a given immune response [157]. Increased prostaglandin E2 production by HIV-infected human macrophages induces apoptosis in co-cultured non-infected lymphocytes [93]. Infection with HIV in vitro leads to increased expression of FasL on monocytes, which leads to cell death of co-cultured uninfected lymphocytes [6].

In conclusion, we propose that, as in other acute non-persistent viral infections, PCD in acute HIV infection is a reflection of immune activation. The increased numbers of cells dying during the asymptomatic phase might be the result of continuous activation priming for death. Although PCD in early asymptomatic infection is merely reflecting the activated immune system rather than being a dominant pathogenic mechanism, virus-induced apoptosis might contribute to CD4+ cell depletion. First by infection of precursor cells or accessory cells affecting the renewal of the T cell compartment and, secondly, when the viral burden increases in late stages directly by HIV-induced apoptosis of peripheral CD4+ T cells.

Biological variation of HIV

One feature of HIV-1 is its great variability with respect to biological properties such as replication rate and cytotropism [4, 29, 49, 146, 152]. The HIV-1 biological phenotype is believed to be an important determinant in the variable clinical course of the infection. The asymptomatic phase of HIV-1 infection is characterized by low frequencies of infected cells in peripheral blood [39, 74], and the predominant HIV-1 variants replicate both in primary T cells and macrophages and are non-syncytium inducing (NSI) [135]. HIV-1-infected macrophages in the tissue compartment are believed to be the viral reservoir because peripheral blood T cells, in the asymptomatic phase of infection, carry preferentially macrophage-tropic viruses compatible with recent infection of these T cells by HIV-1 derived from macrophages [134, 135].

Virus phenotype and kinetics of CD4+ T cell loss

Several groups have analyzed the kinetics of CD4+ T cell counts in progression to AIDS [73, 90, 132, 147]. These studies all showed that between 18 and 24 months before onset of AIDS, CD4+ T cell counts rapidly decline, often paralleled by CD8+ T cell counts. It has been shown that this precipitous drop in CD4+ T cell counts is strongly associated with SI variants and is much less pronounced in patients that develop AIDS with NSI variants [73, 125, 132]. This suggests that SI variants and to some extent late stage NSI variants induce progressively increasing CD4+ T cell turnover and rapid collapse of the immune system. It has been suggested that this could be due to progressive exhaustion of CD4+ T cell renewal.

These SI variants in general are absent in the asymptomatic phase of infection. Since macrophages are the main target cells for the virus to enter upon transmission [120, 150], in the first phase of infection only NSI variants are present and a period of time is needed to generate the specific mutations correlated with the SI phenotype [53, 54]. Until now it is not understood why it takes so long to generate these mutants and why this only happens in a fraction of infected individuals.

SI are escape variants from HIV-1-suppressive chemokines

An interesting component of host immunity that has been ascribed an important role in AIDS pathogenesis is the non-cytolytic inhibition of virus replication by CD8+ T lymphocytes in a major histocompatibility complex class I non-restricted way [18, 127, 161]. Inhibition has been demonstrated to be mediated at least in part by a soluble factor [83, 154, 155]. This suppressive activity has been demonstrated in CD8+ T cells from both HIV-1-positive and -negative individuals as well as from non-human primates [19, 24, 25, 46, 68, 156]. In addition, CD8+ lymphocytes from long-term asymptomatic HIV-1-infected individuals show vigorous HIV-1 suppressive activity and from most of these individuals infectious virus can only be isolated after CD8+ T cell depletion [22]. Next to these CD8+ T cell-derived factors, two groups recently reported cloning of HIV inhibitory factors, revealing its identities as IL-16 in one report [7] and as a combination of RANTES, MIP-1α and MIP-1β in another [37]. Cocchi et al. [37] showed that these chemokines acted predominantly on laboratory adapted, so-called SI non-macrophage tropic isolates. Paxton et al. [122] described two patients that appeared to have CD4+ T cells insusceptible to infection with primary macrophage tropic NSI isolates and the CD4+ T cells of both patients produced high amounts of the three chemokines. The patients cells could be readily infected with SI primary isolates, suggesting that the chemokines did not inhibit SI variants. To us, this all suggests that in early infection the predominant viruses present are NSI that are sensitive to inhibition and control by the three chemokines, but during the course of infection, SI variants emerge that have become insensitive to inhibition by RANTES, MIP-1α and MIP-1β. Indeed studies from our laboratory have shown relative insensitivity of SI viruses compared to NSI viruses isolated from a single individual to CD8+-derived inhibitory factors (Kootstra et al., submitted for publication). This indicates that SI variants have to be seen as escape variants from immune pressure, initially RANTES but later on from other inhibitory factors as well.

Altered T cell function and cytokine network

Already prior to the loss of CD4$^+$ T cells in later stages of infection, HIV-1 infection is characterized by functional defects of T cells in vitro, which are observed from early infection on. Proliferation of T cells in response to ligation of the TCR/CD3 complex is impaired [8, 58, 100, 138] and IL-2 production decreased [32, 62]. In addition, delayed-type hypersensitivity (DTH) reactions are decreased in vivo [14, 91]. In our view this early imune dysfunction is instrumental in paving the way for the virus to be ultimately capable of inducing immune collapse and severe immune deficiency [101].

The fact that both CD4$^+$ and CD8$^+$ T cells of HIV-1-infected individuals are disturbed in their function [62, 100] in a stage of infection where the number of infected T cells is low [133], asks for a systemic explanation for the observed T cell dysfunction. When T cell dysfunction in HIV-1-infected individuals is studied in detail, it is clear that functional properties ascribed to Th1 cells are specifically disturbed. Since 1993 when Clerici and Shearer [30] proposed that T cell dysfunction in HIV-1 infection was associated with a change in cytokines secreted by Th cells from Th1 to Th2 cells, many studies on cytokine secretion patterns of T cells from HIV-1-infected individuals have been reported.

Dysregulated cytokine patterns in HIV-1 infection

One approach to study the capacity of patient T cells to secrete a certain cytokine is to generate T cell clones. Maggi et al. [84] reported already in 1987 a reduced number of T cell clones producing IL-2 and interferon (IFN)-γ in AIDS patients. Recently, the same group generated a large panel of CD4$^+$ T cell clones specific for purified protein derivative of tuberculin or *Toxoplasma gondii* and observed a significant increase in the production of Th2 cytokines by clones generated from HIV-1-infected individuals, resulting in an increased percentage of Th0 type clones [86]. In agreement with this, T cell clones generated by random cloning procedures from CD4$^+$ memory cells from asymptomatically HIV-1-infected individuals comprised increased numbers of Th0 clones [96]. In addition to this increased percentage of Th0/Th2 CD4$^+$ T cell clones, CD8$^+$ T cell lines and clones have been generated from symptomatic HIV-1-infected individuals that can provide helper activity for IgE synthesis [118] and show decreased cytolytic activity [85]. These CD8$^+$ T cells indeed have Th2-like cytokine secretion patterns [85, 118].

Next to analyses of T cell lines and T cell clones, studies on cytokine production after stimulation of PBMC in vitro have been published. Decreased IL-2 production by T cells from HIV-1-infected individuals in vitro has been extensively documented [10, 33, 51, 56, 69, 99, 166]. However, for other Th1 and Th2 cytokines, conflicting results have been reported. A clear-cut shift to Th2 responses in bulk cultures, has so far only been reported by Clerici et al. [30], who showed a decreased IL-2 production induced by recall antigen but an increased mitogen-induced IL-4 production by PBMC from HIV-1-infected individuals in certain phases of infection. Autran et al. [5] described a specific subset of CD4$^+$ T cells, lacking CD7 expression, which have a Th2-like cytokine secretion pattern and are increased in number in HIV-1-infected individuals. However, increased IL-4 production as reported by Clerici et al. [30] has only been reported by two other groups [69, 110], while most reports show unchanged [44, 45, 113, 166] or decreased [10, 42, 48, 86, 99] IL-4 production. It should be noted that most studies on PBMC cultures show a general decrease of all cytokines studied, probably due to the fact that T cells from HIV-1-infected individuals respond less well to a polyclonal T cell activation signal in vitro [10, 86, 99]. Thus, in agreement with a decrease in Th1 cytokine secretion, decreased IFN-γ production was published in very early [108, 109] and more recent studies [10, 56, 69, 99, 166]. On the other hand, increased IFN-γ production, probably originating from mainly CD8$^+$ T cells, and possibly reflecting activated cellular immunity, has been reported [45, 51, 60, 110, 153].

IL-10, a clear Th2 cytokine in mice, is produced in humans by both Th1- and Th2-type T cells [163], but might be considered 'Th2' because of its immunosuppressive effects [31]. IL-10 can be produced by different cell types, which may explain the conflicting data on IL-10 production in HIV-1 infection reported so far. In line with other monokines, the increase in IL-10 production in HIV-1-infected individuals [10, 36, 41, 51, 60] might be due to production by mainly monocytes [45]. Unresponsiveness of T cells might be the cause of the observation that IL-10 production is decreased or unaltered in other studies [28, 42, 48, 99, 166].

One should keep in mind that the various results on cytokine secretion in HIV-1-infected individuals might be related to the stage of infection of the patients studied, in addition to differences in cell preparations, mode of activation of cells and, not least, in cytokine assays. Furthermore, one must be careful in comparing data on cytokine responsiveness obtained by T cell cloning with results of bulk PBMC cultures. By generating T cell clones the potential of T cells to secrete a certain cytokine is studied under optimal circumstances. By analyzing PBMC stimulated in bulk, the intrinsic decreased responses to the stimulus by cells from HIV-1-infected subjects might bias the observation as to whether the cells have a commitment in vivo to secrete a certain cytokine. Furthermore, cross-regulation of different cell types in bulk cultures might influence the outcome. Single-cell analysis of cytokine secretion by T cells from HIV-1-infected individuals gives insight in the number of cells that are capable of producing either IFN-γ or IL-4, regardless the amount of cytokines they are producing. Indeed, on single-cell analysis by intracellular staining, we observed a significant decrease in the ratio of cells producing IFN-γ and IL-4 in HIV-1-infected individuals, in agreement with the findings in T cell clones [99].

The conclusion from our data and those discussed here might be that there is a decrease in Th1-type cytokine production causing a disturbance of the balance between Th1 and Th2 responses, leading to a Th0-like cytokine profile. In view of this, cytokines produced by APC that are critical for polarization of Th cell responses are of interest. The main cytokines in this context are IL-10 and IL-12. Since IL-10 can be produced by different cell types, including T cells, this cytokine has been discussed in the previous paragraph. IL-12 plays a critical role in Th1 cell differentiation [67]. Chehimi et al. [28] were the first to publish that PBMC from HIV-1-infected individuals are impaired in IL-12 p40 and p70 production upon stimulation with *Staphylococcus aureus* antigen (SAC). A similar finding was obtained with stimulation with *T. gondii* antigen for IL-12 p40 [56]. Alveolar macrophages from asymptomatically infected individuals, however, produce increased amounts of IL-12 p70 when stimulated with bacterial antigens and a decreased IL-12 secretion was only found in patients with AIDS [41]. In a whole blood culture system, we demonstrated decreased IL-12 p40 and p70 production upon SAC but not lipopolysaccharide stimulation in HIV-infected persons. No relation with IL-10 or prostaglandin E2, potential inhibitors of IL-12 production, was found in these individuals [98]. These results at this time are suggestive of an underlying failure to produce the required amount of IL-12 to mount proper Th1 responses.

Cytokines and immune modulation

Proliferative responses to recall antigen are already disturbed early in HIV-1 infection and can be restored in vitro by IL-2 [80, 138]. IL-2 is also capable of restoring HIV-1-specific proliferative responses in vitro [11, 137]. In addition, the recently described IL-2-like cytokine IL-15 seems to have similar and synergistic effects to IL-2 on T cell proliferation from HIV-1-infected individuals and controls [137].

In recent years, in view of the publications on Th1/Th2 cytokine disturbances, in vitro manipulation of proliferative responses by various cytokines or anti-cytokines antibodies has been widely studied. IL-12 is capable of enhancing proliferation of T cells from HIV-1-infected individuals in response to influenza, HIV-1 peptides [34], *Mycobacterium avium* [112, 137] and polyclonal T cell stimulators [137]. Furthermore IFN-γ production in response to several T cell stimulators in vitro is enhanced upon IL-12 addition [34, 137, 166]. When T cells from HIV-1-infected individuals are cloned in the presence of IL-12, an increased outgrowth of IFN-γ-producing cells is observed [119]. Thus, IL-12 seems capable of restoring T cell defects in vitro. However, it should be noted that in most publications it was reported that T cells from non-infected controls are also enhanced in their proliferative responses and IFN-γ production in the presence of IL-12 [112, 137]. The enhanced outgrowth of IFN-γ-producing T cells in the presence of IL-12 is also observed when T cells from non-infected controls are used [88, 89, 119, 164]. This suggests that IL-12 does not restore a disturbed balance, but, at least in vitro, just enhances Th1-mediated responses, which is also observable in normal conditions. In agreement with this, a general enhancing effect of IL-12 on natural killer cell function was observed in both HIV-1-infected individuals and controls [27].

IL-10 has also been implied to play a major role in HIV-1-induced immune deficiency. Indeed, addition of neutralizing antibodies to T cell cultures enhances proliferative responses [36, 166]. In the original studies by Clerici et al. [33], neutralizing anti-IL-4 mAb were shown to be capable of restoring proliferative responses, but seemed to be much less efficient than anti-IL-10 antibodies [36].

Since T cells from HIV-1-infected individuals are impaired in their capacity to produce IL-2, needed for intact T cell proliferative responses, suppletion with IL- 2 would be a logical form of immune therapy in HIV-1-infected individuals. Indeed, several studies on IL-2 therapy have been published in the last few years, all in individuals that were simultaneously treated with anti-viral drugs, in most cases zidovudine. Low-dose IL-2 treatment was demonstrated in several studies to increase immune functions, especially in individuals with higher CD4$^+$ T cell counts, without increases in viral load [143, 144, 162]. Prolonged treatment with IL-2 recently demonstrated beneficial effects in individuals with CD4$^+$ T cell counts above 200/mm^3, while patients with less $CD4^+$ T cells showed little immunological improvement but did show evidence of increased viral activation and suffered from toxic effects [76].

Another candidate for immune therapy is IFN-α, not primarily because of its immune modulatory potential but because of its anti-viral capacities [57]. IFN-α is produced in increased amounts during natural HIV-1 infection, and resistance to IFN-α of HIV-1 variants was demonstrated in the course of infection. Thus, it was proposed that IFN-α therapy would only be useful in early stages of HIV-1 infection [57]. A phase I trial of IFN-α in combination with IL-2 showed few side effects and preliminary evidence for immune modulation and anti-viral activity [55]. IFN-α together with zidovudine had beneficial, though transient, effects on $CD4^+$ T cell numbers and T cell function when compared with zidovudine alone [55].

Recently, IL-12 has been greeted enthusiastically as a potential immune modulator to administer to HIV-1-infected individuals [63]. Although single-dose treatment induced little or no adverse effects, in clinical trials in cancer patients, repetitive infusions inducing episodes of severe toxicity have been reported, which points to caution in using IL-12 as a therapeutic agent [38]. Furthermore, although there are many reports on beneficial effects of IL-12 in animal models of parasitic and bacterial infections, there is still relatively little known of the effects on IL-12 on viral infections in animal models. Whereas low-dose treatment with IL-12 is capable of enhancing the cellular immune response against LCMV infection in mice, high-dose IL-12 treatment results in enhanced virus burden in these animals [114]. IL-12-mediated cytotoxicity in these high-dose IL-12 treated animals might be explained by the increased production of tumor necrosis factor (TNF)-α upon IL-12 treatment [115]. In addition, in human T cells IL-12 is capable of inducing the production of the immunosuppressive cytokine IL-10 in vitro [97]. Thus, prolonged IL-12 treatment might lead to immunosuppression due to increased production of cytokines as TNF-α and IL-10 and lead to an increased viral burden and failure of the immune system to prevent this.

Concluding remarks

The rationale behind immune modulation in HIV-1 infected individuals should not only be correction of cytokines that are over- or underproduced in the course of infection. To estimate the chance of success of immune modulation in vivo, a more basic question has to be answered first: how important is the gradual loss of cellular immunity in immunopathogenesis of HIV-1 infection? One may reason that with a properly functioning immune system, HIV-1 will never get the chance to give rise to overt virus replication and severe $CD4^+$ T cell loss. Some findings indeed make a case for an important role of the failing immune system in progression to AIDS. First, the loss of T cell function is predictive for rapid progression to AIDS independent from $CD4^+$ T cell numbers [66, 126, 131] and, secondly, in individuals who remain asymptomatic for a prolonged period of time, immune function is preserved [71, 139].

To understand the role of a deteriorating immune system in AIDS pathogenesis, many questions remain to be answered, one of the most important being the contribution to protection from disease made by cytotoxic T lymphocytes (CTL) [100]. There is some controversy as to the role of HIV-1-specific CTL in controlling virus infection [167]. Studies in long-term asymptomatic individuals have demonstrated preserved HIV-1 gag-specific CTL responses [72], suggestive of a contribution in controlling virus load. However, despite the presence of strong CTL responses, viral load did increase in people who progressed rapidly to AIDS [72]. Based on these results, one may conclude that HIV-1-specific CTL do not play a critical role in determining the rate of progression to AIDS. Alternatively, one could argue that in vivo, although in these individuals CTL precursors are present, they are not capable of exerting their function properly. The CTL precursor frequency in this study was determined by limiting dilution culture and propagation of cells under optimal in vitro conditions. Defective presentation of HIV-1 antigens, lack of IL-12 or increased IL-10 production and decreased Th1 responses in vivo may all lead to the failure of cellular immune responses. This would point to an important role for APC and Th cells. Lack of cellular immunity would lead to lack of CTL responses and increasing viral loads. Cellular immunity has even been proposed to be correlated with protection from HIV-1 infection [129], but clear evidence to formally proof this point is lacking [102].

To be able to adequately and successfully intervene by immunotherapy in HIV-1 infection, we need to gain more insight into why the host fails to successfully handle this virus infection. Given the complexity of virus-host interactions, integrated viro-immunological studies are required to determine what the critical event(s) is/are that eventually lead to loss of CD4⁺ T cells and progression to disease in HIV-1-infected individuals [103]. Hopefully, this will lead to the development of therapeutic strategies leading to prevention of disease progression.

References

1. Akbar AN, Borthwick NJ, Salmon M, Gombert W, Bofill M, Shamsadeen N, Pilling D, Pett S, Grundy JE, Janossy G (1993) The significance of low bcl-2 expression by CD45RO T cells in normal individuals and patients with acute viral infections. The role of apoptosis in T cell memory. J Exp Med 178:427
2. Akbar AN, Salmon M, Savill J, Janossy G (1993) A possible role for bcl-2 in regulating T cell memory – a 'balancing act' between cell death and survival. Immunol Today 14:526
3. Ameisen JC, Capron A (1991) Cell dysfunction and depletion in AIDS: the programmed cell death hypothesis. Immunol Today 12:102
4. Asjo B, Albert J, Karlsson A, Morfeldt-Månson L, Biberfeld G, Lidman K, Fenyo EM (1986) Replicative properties of human immunodeficiency virus from patients with varying severity of HIV infection. Lancet II:660
5. Autran B, Legac E, Blanc C, Debré P (1995) A Th0/Th2-like function of CD4⁺CD7⁻ helper cells from normal donors and HIV-infected patients. J Immunol 154:1408
6. Badley AD, McElhinny JA, Leibson PJ, Lynch DH, Alderson MR, Paya CV (1996) Upregulation of Fas ligand expression by human immunodeficiency virus in human macrophages mediates apoptosis of uninfected T lymphocytes. J Virol 70:199
7. Baier M, Werner A, Bannert N, Metzner K, Kurth R (1995) HIV suppression by interleukin-16. Nature 378:563
8. Ballet JJ, Couderc LJ, Rabian-Herzog C, Duval-Roy C, Janier M, Danon F, Clauvel JP, Seligmann M (1988) Impaired T-lymphocyte-dependent immune responses to microbial antigens in patients with HIV-1-associated persistent generalized lymphadenopathy. J Acquir Immune Defic Syndr 2:291
9. Banda NK, Bernier J, Kurahara DK, Kurrle R, Haigwood N, Sekaly R-P, Helman Finkel T (1992) Crosslinking CD4 by human immunodeficiency virus gp120 primes T cells for activation-induced apoptosis. J Exp Med 176:1099
10. Barcellini W, Rizzardi GP, Borghi MO, Fain C, Lazzarin A, Meroni PL (1994) Th1 and Th2 cytokine production by peripheral blood mononuclear cells from HIV-infected patients. J Acquir Immune Defic Syndr 8:757
11. Bell SJD, Cooper DA, Kemp BE, Doherty RR, Penny R (1992) Heterogenous effects of exogenous IL-2 on HIV-specific cell-mediated immunity (CMI). Clin Exp Immunol 90:6

12. Bishop CJ, Moss DJ, Ryan JM, Burrows SR (1985) T lymphocytes in infectious mononucleosis. II. Response in vitro to interleukin-2 and establishment of T cell lines. Clin Exp Immunol 60:70
13. Bishop SA, Gruffydd-Jones TJ, Harbour DA, Stokes CR (1993) Programmed cell death (apoptosis) as a mechanism of cell death in peripheral blood mononuclear cells from cats infected with feline immunodeficiency virus (FIV). Clin Exp Immunol 93:65
14. Blatt SP, Hendrix CW, Butzin CA, Freeman TM, Ward WW, Hensley RE, Melcher GP, Donovan DJ, Boswell RN (1993) Delayed type hypersensitivity skin testing predicts progression to AIDS in HIV-infected patients. Ann Intern Med 119:177
15. Bofill M, Gombert W, Borthwick NJ, Akbar AN, McLaughlin JE, Lee CA, Johnson MA, Pinching AJ, Janossy G (1995) Presence of $CD3^+CD8^+Bcl-2^{low}$ lymphocytes udergoing apoptosis and activated macrophages in lymph nodes of $HIV-1^+$ patients. Am J Pathol 146:1542
16. Bonyhadi ML, Rabin L, Salimi S, Brown DA, Kosek J, McCune JM, Kaneshima H (1993) HIV induces thymus depletion in vivo. Nature 363:728
17. Boudet F, Lecoeur H, Gougeon M (1996) Apoptosis associated with ex vivo down-regulation of Bcl-2 and upregulation of Fas in potential cytotoxic $CD8^+$ T lymphocytes during HIV-1 infection. J Immunol 156:2282
18. Brinchmann JE, Gaudernack G, Vartal F (1990) $CD8^+$ T cells inhibit HIV replication in naturally infected $CD4^+$ T cells. J Immunol 144:2961
19. Brinchmann JE, Gaudernack G, Vartdal F (1990) $CD8^+$ T cells inhibit HIV replication in naturally infected $CD4^+$ T cells. Evidence for a soluble inhibitor. J Immunol 146:2961
20. Buttke TM, Sandstrom PA (1994) Oxidative stress as a mediator of apoptosis. Immunol Today 15:7
21. Cameron PU, Pope M, Gezelter S, Steinman RM (1994) Infection and apoptotic cell death of $CD4^+$ T cells during an immune response to HIV-1 pulsed dendritic cells. AIDS Res Hum Retroviruses 10:61
22. Cao Y, Qin L, Zhang L, Safrit JT, Ho DD (1995) Virologic and immunologic characterization of long-term survivors of Human Immunodeficiency Virus type 1 infection. N Engl J Med 332:201
23. Carbonari M, Cibati M, Pesce AM, Sbarigia D, Grossi P, D'Offizi G, Luzi G, Fiorilli M (1995) Frequency of provirus-bearing $CD4^+$ cells in HIV type 1 infection correlates with extent of in vitro apoptosis of $CD8^+$ but not of $CD4^+$ cells. AIDS Res Hum Retroviruses 11:789
24. Castro BA, Walker CM, Eichberg JW, Levy JA (1991) Suppression of human immunodeficiency virus replication by $CD8^+$ cells from infected and uninfected chimpanzees. Cell Immunol 132:246
25. Castro BA, Homsy J, Lennette E, Murthy KK, Eichberg JW, Levy JA (1992) HIV-1 expression in chimpanzees can be activated by $CD8^+$ cell depletion or CMV infection. Clin Immunol Immunopathol 65:227
26. Cefai D, Debre P, Kaczorek M, Idziorek T, Autran B, Bismuth G (1990) Human immunodeficiency virus-1 glycoproteins gp120 and gp160 specifically inhibit the CD3/T cell-antigen receptor phospho-inositide transduction pathway. J Clin Invest 86:2117
27. Chehimi J, Starr SE, Frank I, Rengaraju M, Jackson SJ, Llanes C, Kobayashi M, Perussia B, Young D, Nickbarg E, Wolf SF, Trinchieri G (1992) Natural killer (NK) cell stimulatory factor increases the cytotoxic activity of NK cells from both healthy donors and human immunodeficiency virus-infected patients. J Exp Med 175:789
28. Chehimi J, Starr SE, Frank I, D'Andrea A, Ma X, MacGregor RR, Sennelier J, Trinchieri G (1994) Impaired interleukin 12 production in human immunodeficiency virus infected patients. J Exp Med 179:1361
29. Cheng-Mayer C, Seto D, Tateno M, Levy JA (1988) Biologic features of HIV-1 that correlate with virulence in the host. Science 240:80
30. Clerici M, Shearer GM (1993) A $T_H1 \rightarrow T_H2$ switch is a critical step in the etiology of HIV infection. Immunol Today 14:107
31. Clerici M, Shearer GM (1994) The Th1-Th2 hypothesis of HIV infection: new insights. Immunol Today 15:575
32. Clerici M, Via CS, Lucey DR, Roilides E, Pizzo PA, Shearer GM (1991) Functional dichotomy of $CD4^+$ T helper lymphocytes in asymptomatic human immunodeficiency virus infection. Eur J Immunol 21:665
33. Clerici M, Hakim FT, Venzon DJ, Blatt S, Hendrix CW, Wynn TA, Shearer GM (1993) Changes in interleukin-2 and interleukin-4 production in asymptomatic human immunodeficiency virus-seropositive individuals. J Clin Invest 91:759

34. Clerici M, Lucey DR, Berzofsky JA, Pinto LA, Wynn TA, Blatt SP, Dolan MJ, Hendrix CW, Wolf SF, Shearer GM (1993) Restoration of HIV- specific cell-mediated immune responses by interleukin-12 in vitro. Science 262:1721
35. Clerici M, Sarin A, Coffman RL, Wynn TA, Blatt SP, Hendrix CW, Wolf SF, Shearer GM, Henkart PA (1994) Type 1/type 2 cytokine modulation of T cell programed cell death as a model for human immunodeficiency virus pathogenesis. Proc Natl Acad Sci USA 91:11811
36. Clerici M, Wynn TA, Berzofsky JA, Blatt SP, Hendrix CW, Sher A, Coffman RL, Shearer GM (1994) Role of interleukin-10 (IL-10) in T helper cell dysfunction in asymptomatic individuals infected with the human immunodeficiency virus (HIV-1). J Clin Invest 93:768
37. Cocchi F, DeVico AL, Garzino-Demo A, Arya SK, Gallo RC, Lusso P (1995) Identification of RANTES, MIP-1α, and MIP-1β as the major HIV-suppressive factors produced by CD8$^+$ T cells. Science 270:1811
38. Cohen J (1995) Clinical trials. IL-12 deaths: explanation and a puzzle. Science 270:908
39. Connor RI, Mohri H, Cao Y, Ho DD (1993) Increased viral burden and cytopathicity correlate temporally with CD4$^+$ T-lymphocyte decline and clinical progression in human immunodeficiency virus type 1 infected infected individuals. J Virol 67:1772
40. Critchfield JM, Racke MK, Zúñiga-Pflücker JC, Cannella B, Raine CS, Goverman J, Lenardo MJ (1994) T cell deletion in high antigen dose therapy of autoimmune encephalomyelitis. Science 263:1139
41. Denis M, Ghadirian E (1994) Dysregulation of interleukin 8, interleukin 10, and interleukin 12 release by alveolar macrophages from HIV type 1-infected subjects. AIDS Res Hum Retroviruses 10:1619
42. Diaz-Mitoma F, Kumar A, Karimi S, Kryworuchko M, Daftarian MP, Creery WD, Filion LG, Cameron W (1995) Expression of IL-10, IL-4 and interferon-gamma in unstimulated and mitogen-stimulated peripheral blood lymphocytes from HIV-seropositive patients. Clin Exp Immunol 102:31
43. Dröge W, Eck HP, Mihm S (1992) HIV-induced cysteine deficiency and T cell dysfunction – a rationale for treatment with N-acetylcysteine. Immunol Today 13:211
44. Eckwalanga M, Marussig M, Dias Tavares M, Bouanga JC, Hulier E, Pavlovitch JH, Minoprio P, Portnoi D, Rénia L, Mazier D (1994) Murine AIDS protects mice against experimental cerebral malaria: down-regulation by interleukin 10 of a T-helper type 1 CD4$^+$ cell-mediated pathology. Proc Natl Acad Sci USA 91:8097
45. Emilie D, Fior R, Llorente L, Marfaing-Koka A, Peuchmaur M, Devergne O, Jarousse B, Wijdenes J, Boue F, Galanaud P (1994) Cytokines from lymphoid organs of HIV-infected patients: production and role in the immune disequilibrium of the disease and in the development of B lymphomas. Immunol Rev 140:5
46. Ennen J, Findeklee H, Dittmar MT, Norley S, Ernst M, Kurth R (1994) CD8$^+$ T lymphocytes of african green monkeys secrete an immunodeficiency virus-suppressing lymphokine. Proc Natl Acad Sci USA 91:7207
47. Estaquier J, Idziorek T, De Bels F, Barré-Sinoussi F, Hurtrel B, Aubertin A-M, Venet A, Mehtali M, Muchmore E, Michel P, Mouton Y, Girard M, Ameisen JC (1994) Programmed cell death and AIDS: Significance of T cell apoptosis in pathogenic and nonpathogenic primate lentiviral infections. Proc Natl Acad Sci USA 91:9431
48. Estaquier J, Idziorek T, Zou W, Emilie D, Farber C-M, Bourez J- M, Ameisen JC (1995) T helper type 1/T helper type 2 cytokines and T cell death: preventive effect of interleukin 12 on activation-induced and CD95 (FAS/APO- 1)-mediated apoptosis of CD4$^+$ T cells from human immunodeficency virus- infected persons. J Exp Med 182:1759
49. Evans LA, McHugh TM, Stites DP, Levy JA (1987) Differential ability of HIV isolates to productively infect human cells. J Immunol 138:3415
50. Eyster ME, Gail MH, Ballard JO, Al-Mondiry H, Goedert JJ (1987) Natural history of human im-munodeficiency virus infections in hemophiliacs: effects of T cell subsets, platelet counts, and age. Ann Intern Med 107:1
51. Fan J, Bass HZ, Fahey JL (1993) Elevated IFN-gamma and decreased IL-2 gene expression are associated with HIV infection. J Immunol 151:5031
52. Finkel TH, Tudor-Williams G, Banda NK, Cotton MF, Curiel T, Monks C, Baba TW, Ruprecht RM, Kupfer A (1995) Apoptosis occurs predominantly in bystander cells and not in productively infected cells of HIV- and SIV-infected lymph nodes. Nature Med 1:129

53. Fouchier RAM, Groenink M, Kootstra NA, Tersmette M, Huisman HG, Miedema F, Schuitemaker H (1992) Phenotype-associated sequence variation in the third variable domain of the human immunodeficiency virus type 1 gp120 molecule. J Virol 66:3183

54. Fouchier RAM, Broersen SM, Brouwer M, Tersmette M, Van 't Wout AB, Groenink M, Schuitemaker H (1995) Temporal relationship between elongation of the HIV-1 gp120 V2 domain and the conversion towards a syncytium inducing phenotype. AIDS Res Hum Retroviruses 11:1473

55. Frissen PHJ, Van der Ende ME, Ten Napel CHH, Weigel HM, Schreij GS, Kauffmann RH, Koopmans PP, Hoepelman AIM, De Boer JB, Weverling GJ, Haverkamp G, Dowd P, Miedema F, Schuurman R, Boucher CAB, Lange JMA (1994) Zidovudine and interferon-α combination therapy versus zidovudine monotherapy in subjects with symptomatic human immunodeficiency virus type 1 infection. J Infect Dis 169:1351

56. Gazzinelli RT, Bala S, Stevens R, Baseler M, Wahl L, Kovacs J, Sher A (1995) HIV infection suppresses type 1 lymphokine and IL-12 responses to *Toxoplasma gondii* but fails to inhibit the synthesis of other parasite-induced monokines. J Immunol 155:1565

57. Gendelman HE, Baldwin T, Baca-Regen L, Swindells S, Loomis L, Skurkovich S (1994) Regulation of HIV1 replication by interferon alpha: from laboratory bench to bedside. Res Immunol 145:679

58. Giorgi JV, Fahey JL, Smith DC, Hultin LE, Cheng HL, Mitsuyasu RT, Detels R (1987) Early effects of HIV on CD4 lymphocytes in vivo. J Immunol 138:3725

59. Gougeon M, Garcia S, Heeney J, Tschopp R, Lecoeur H, Guetard D, Rame V, Dauguet R, Montagnier L (1993) Programmed cell death in AIDS- related HIV and SIV infections. AIDS Res Hum Retroviruses 9:553

60. Graziosi C, Pantaleo G, Gantt KR, Fortin J-P, Demarest JF, Cohen OJ, Sékaly RF, Fauci AS (1994) Lack of evidence for the dichotomy of Th1 and Th2 predominance in HIV-infected individuals. Science 265:248

61. Groux H, Torpier G, Monté D, Mouton Y, Capron A, Ameisen JC (1992) Activation-induced death by apoptosis in CD4+ T cells from human immunodeficiency virus-infected asymptomatic individuals. J Exp Med 175:331

62. Gruters RA, Terpstra FG, De Jong R, Van Noesel CJM, Van Lier RAW, Miedema F (1990) Selective loss of T cell functions in different stages of HIV infection. Eur J Immunol 20:1039

63. Hall SS (1994) IL-12 holds promise against cancer, glimmer of AIDS hope. Science 263:1685

64. Ho DD, Neumann AU, Perelson AS, Chen W, Leonard JM, Markowitz M (1995) Rapid turnover of plasma virions and CD4 lymphocytes in HIV-1 infection. Nature 373:123

65. Ho DD, Perelson AS, Shaw GM (1995) HIV results in the frame (Reply). Nature 375:198

66. Hofmann B, Orskov Lindhardt B, Gerstoft J, Sand Petersen C, Platz P, Ryder LP, Odum N, Dickmeiss E, Nielsen PB, Ullman S, Svejgaard A (1987) Lymphocyte transformation response to pokeweed mitogen as a marker for the development of AIDS and AIDS related symptoms in homosexual men with HIV antibodies. Br Med J 295:293

67. Hsieh C-S, Macatonia SE, Tripp CS, Wolf ST, O'Gara A, Murphy KM (1993) Development of Th1 CD4+ T cells through IL-12 produced by Listeria-induced macrophages. Science 260:547

68. Hsueh FW, Walker CM, Blackbourn DJ, Levy JA (1994) Suppression of HIV replication by CD8+ cell clones derived from HIV-infected and uninfected individuals. Cell Immunol 159:271

69. Hyjek E, Lischner HW, Hyslop T, Bartkowiak J, Kubin M, Trinchieri G, Kozbor D (1995) Cytokine patterns during progression to AIDS in children with perinatal HIV infection. J Immunol 155:4060

70. Katsikis PD, Wunderlich ES, Smith CA, Herzenberg LA, Herzenberg L (1995) Fas antigen stimulation induces marked apoptosis of T lymphocytes in human immunodeficiency virus-infected individuals. J Exp Med 181:2029

71. Keet IPM, Krol A, Klein MR, Veugelers P, De Wit J, Roos MTL, Koot M, Goudsmit J, Miedema F, Coutinho RA (1994) Characteristics of long- term asymptomatic infection with the human immunodeficiency virus Type 1 with normal and low CD4+ cell counts. J Infect Dis 169:1236

72. Klein MR, van Baalen CA, Holwerda AM, Kerkhof-Garde SR, Bende RJ, Keet IPM, Eeftinck Schattenkerk JKM, Osterhaus ADME, Schuitemaker H, Miedema F (1995) Kinetics of Gag-specific CTL responses during the clinical course of HIV-1 infection: a longitudinal analysis of rapid progressors and long-term asymptomatics. J Exp Med 181:1365

73. Koot M, Keet IPM, Vos AHV, De Goede REY, Roos MThL, Coutinho RA, Miedema F, Schellekens PThA, Tersmette M (1993) Prognostic value of human immunodeficiency virus type 1 biological phenotype for rate of CD4+ cell depletion and progression to AIDS. Ann Intern Med 118:681

74. Koot M, Van 't Wout AB, Kootstra NA, De Goede REY, Tersmette M, Schuitemaker H (1996) Relation between changes in cellular load, evolution of viral phenotype, and the clonal composition of virus populations in the course of human immunodeficiency virus type 1 infection. J Infect Dis 173:349

75. Korsmeyer SJ (1992) Bcl-2: a repressor of lymphocyte death. Immunol Today 13:285

76. Kovacs JA, Baseler M, Dewar RJ, Vogel S, Davey RT Jr, Falloon J, Polis MA, Walker RE, Stevens R, Salzman NP, Metcalf JA, Masur H, Lane HC (1995) Increases in CD4 T lymphocytes with intermittent courses of interleukin-2 in patients with human immunodeficiency virus infection. N Engl J Med 332:567

77. Laurent-Crawford AG, Krust B, Muller S, Rivière Y, Rey-Cuillé MA, Béchet J-M, Montagnier L, Hovanessian AG (1991) The cytopathic effect of HIV is associated with apoptosis. Virology 185:829

78. Lewis DE, Ng Tang DS, Adu-Oppong A, Schober W, Rodgers JR (1994) Anergy and apoptosis in CD8$^+$ T cells from HIV-infected individuals. J Immunol 153:412

79. Li CJ, Friedman DJ, Wang C, Metelev V, Pardee AB (1995) Induction of apoptosis in uninfected lymphocytes by HIV-1 Tat protein. Science 268:429

80. Lifson JD, Benike CJ, Mark DF, Koths K, Engleman EG (1984) Human recombinant interleukin-2 partly reconstitutes deficient in vitro immune responses of lymphocytes from patients with AIDS. Lancet I:698

81. Lu Y-Y, Koga Y, Tanaka K, Sasaki M, Kimura G, Nomoto K (1994) Apoptosis induced in CD4$^+$ cells expressing gp160 of human immunodeficiency virus type 1. J Virol 68:390

82. Macho A, Castedo M, Marchetti P, Aguilar JJ, Decaudin D, Zamzami N, Girard PM, Uriel J, Kroemer G (1995) Mitochondrial dysfunctions in circulating T lymphocytes from human immunodeficiency virus-1 carriers. Blood 86:2481

83. Mackewicz CE, Yang LC, Lifson JD, Levy JA (1994) Non-cytolytic CD8 T cell anti-HIV responses in primary HIV-1 infection. Lancet 344:1671

84. Maggi E, Macchia D, Parronchi P, Mazzetti M, Ravina A, Milo D, Romagnani S (1987) Reduced production of interleukin-2 and interferon-gamma and enhanced helper activity for IgG synthesis by cloned CD4$^+$ T cells from patients with AIDS. Eur J Immunol 17:1685

85. Maggi E, Giudizi MG, Biagiotti R, Annunziato F, Manetti R, Piccinni M-P, Parronchi P, Sampognaro S, Giannarini L, Zuccati G, Romagnani S (1994) Th2-like CD8$^+$ T cells showing B cell helper function and reduced cytolytic activity in human immunodeficiency virus type 1 infection. J Exp Med 180:489

86. Maggi E, Mazzetti M, Ravina A, Annunziato F, De Carli M, Pesce AM, Del Prete G, Romagnani S (1994) Ability of HIV to promote a Th1 to Th0 shift and to replicate preferentially in Th2 and Th0 cells. Science 265:244

87. Manca F, Habeshaw JA, Dalgleish AG (1990) HIV envelope glycoprotein, antigen specific T cell responses, and soluble CD4. Lancet 335:811

88. Manetti R, Parronchi P, Giudizi MG, Piccinni M-P, Maggi E, Trinchieri G, Romagnani S (1993) Natural killer cell stimulatory factor (interleukin 12 [IL-12]) induces T helper type 1 (Th1)-specific immune responses and inhibits the development of IL-4-producing Th cells. J Exp Med 177:1199

89. Manetti R, Gerosa F, Giudizi M-G, Biagiotti R, Parronchi P, Piccinni M-P, Sampognaro S, Maggi E, Romagnani S, Trinchieri G (1994) Interleukin-12 induces stable priming for interferon-gamma (IFN-gamma) production during differentiation of human T helper (Th) cells and transient IFN-gamma production in established Th2 cell clones. J Exp Med 179:1273

90. Margolick JB, Muñoz A, Donnenberg AD, PARK LP, Galai N, Giorgi JV, O'Gorman MRG, Ferbas J, for the Multicenter AIDS Cohort Study (1995) Failure of T cell homeostasis preceding AIDS in HIV-1 infection. Nature Med 1:674

91. Markowitz N, Hansen NI, Wilcosky TC, Hopewell PC, Glassroth J, Kvale PA, Mangura BT, Osmond D, Wallace JM, Rosen MJ, Reichman LB (1993) Tuberculin and anergy testing in HIV-seropositive and HIV-seronegative persons. Ann Intern Med 119:185

92. Martin SJ, Matear PM, Vyakarnam A (1994) HIV-1 infection of human CD4$^+$ T cells in vitro. Differential induction of apoptosis in these cells. J Immunol 152:330

93. Mastino A, Grelli S, Piacentini M, Oliverio S, Favalli C, Perno CF, Garaci E (1993) Correlation between induction of lymphocyte apoptosis and prostaglandin E2 production by macrophages infected with HIV. Cell Immunol 152:120

94. Meyaard L, Otto SA, Jonker RR, Mijnster MJ, Keet RPM, Miedema F (1992) Programmed death of T cells in HIV-1 infection. Science 257:217

95. Meyaard L, Otto SA, Keet IPM, Roos MThL, Miedema F (1994) Programmed death of T cells in HIV-1 infection: no correlation with progression to disease. J Clin Invest 93:982

96. Meyaard L, Otto SA, Keet IPM, Van Lier RAW, Miedema F (1994) Changes in cytokine secretion patterns of $CD4^+$ T cell clones in HIV-1 infection. Blood 84:4262

97. Meyaard L, Hovenkamp E, Otto SA, Miedema F (1996) IL-12- induced IL-10 production by human T cells as a negative feedback for IL-12- induced immune responses. J Immunol 156:2776

98. Meyaard L, Hovenkamp E, Pakker N, Van der Pouw Kraan TCTM, Miedema F (1996) IL-12 production in whole blood cultures from HIV-infected individuals studied in relation to IL-10 and PGE2 production. Blood (in press)

99. Meyaard L, Hovenkamp E, Keet IPM, Hooibrink B, De Jong IH, Otto SA, Miedema F (1996) Single cell analysis of IL-4 and IFN-gamma production by T cells from HIV infected individuals: decreased IFN-gamma in the presence of preserved IL-4 production. J Immunol (in press)

100. Miedema F, Petit AJC, Terpstra FG, Schattenkerk JKME, De Wolf F, Al BJM, Roos MThL, Lange JMA, Danner SA, Goudsmit J, Schellekens PTA (1988) Immunological abnormalities in human immunodeficiency virus (HIV)-infected asymptomatic homosexual men. HIV affects the immune system before $CD4^+$ T helper cell depletion occurs. J Clin Invest 82:1908

101. Miedema F, Tersmette M, Van Lier RAW (1990) AIDS pathogenesis: a dynamic interaction between HIV and the immune system. Immunol Today 11:293

102. Miedema F, Meyaard L, Klein MR (1993) Protection from HIV-1 infection or AIDS? Science 262:1074

103. Miedema F, Meyaard L, Koot M, Klein MR, Roos MThL, Groenink M, Fouchier RAM, Van 't Wout AB, Tersmette M, Schellekens PThA, Schuitemaker H (1994) Changing virus-host interactions in the course of HIV-1 infection. Immunol Rev 140:35

104. Miyawaki T, Uehara T, Nibu R, Tsuji T, Yachie A, Yonehara S, Taniguchi N (1992) Differential expression of apoptosis-related Fas antigen on lymphocyte subpopulations in human peripheral blood. J Immunol 149:3753

105. Moss AR, Bachetti P, Osmond D, Krampf W, Chaisson RE, Stites D, Wilber J, Allain JP, Carlson J (1988) Seropositivity of HIV and the development of AIDS or AIDS-related conditions: Three year follow-up of the San Francisco General Hospital cohort. Br Med J 269:745

106. Moss DJ, Bishop CJ, Burrows SR, Ryan JM (1985) T lymphocytes in infectious mononucleosis.I.T cell death in vitro. Clin Exp Immunol 60:61

107. Muro-Cacho CA, Pantaleo G, Fauci AS (1995) Analysis of apoptosis in lymph nodes of HIV-infected persons. Intensity of apoptosis correlates with the general state of activation of the lymphoid tissue and not with stage of disease or viral burden. J Immunol 154:5555

108. Murray HW, Hillman JK, Rubin BY, Kelly CD, Jacobs JL, Tyler LW, Donelly DM, Carriero SM, Godbold JH, Roberts RB (1985) Patients at risk for AIDS-related opportunistic infections.Clinical manifestations and impaired gamma interferon production. N Engl J Med 313:1504

109. Murray HW, Scavuzzo DA, Kelly CD, Rubin BY, Roberts RB (1988) $T4^+$ cell production of interferon gamma and the clinical spectrum of patients at risk for and with acquired immunodeficiency syndrome. Arch Intern Med 148:1613

110. Navikas V, Link J, Wahren B, Persson C, Link H (1994) Increased levels of interferon-gamma (IFN-gamma), IL-4 and transforming growth factor-β (TGF-β) mRNA expressing blood mononuclear cells in human HIV infection. Clin Exp Immunol 96:59

111. Newell MK, Haughn LJ, Maroun CR, Julius MH (1990) Death of mature T cells by separate ligation of CD4 and the T cell receptor for antigen. Nature 347:286

112. Newman GW, Guarnaccia JR, Vance III EA, Wu J-Y, Remold HG, Kazanjian PH Jr (1994) Interleukin-12 enhances antigen-specific proliferation of peripheral blood mononuclear cells from HIV-positive and negative donors in response to *Mycobacterium avium*. AIDS 8:1413

113. Nye KE, Knox KA, Pinching AJ (1990) HIV infection of H9 lymphoblastoid cells chronically activates the inositol polyphosphate pathway. AIDS 4:41

114. Orange JS, Wolf SF, Biron CA (1994) Effects of IL-12 on the response and susceptibility to experimental viral infections. J Immunol 152:1253

115. Orange JS, Salazar-Mather TP, Opal SM, Spencer RL, Miller AH, McEwen BS, Biron CA (1995) Mechanism of interleukin 12-mediated toxicities during experimental viral infections: role of tumor necrosis factor and glucocorticoids. J Exp Med 181:901

116. Oyaizu N, Chirmule N, Kalyanaraman VS, Hall WW, Good RA, Pahwa S (1990) Human immunodeficiency virus type 1 envelope glycoprotein gp120 produces immune defects in CD4$^+$ T lymphocytes by inhibiting interleukin 2 mRNA. Proc Natl Acad Sci USA 87:2379

117. Oyaizu N, McCloskey TW, Coronesi M, Chirmule N, Kalyanaraman VS, Pahwa S (1993) Accelerated apoptosis in peripheral blood mononuclear cells (PBMCs) from human immunodeficiency virus type-1 infected patients and in CD4 cross-linked PBMCs from normal individuals. Blood 82:3392

118. Paganelli R, Scala E, Ansotegui IJ, Ausiello CM, Halapi E, Fanales-Belasio E, D'Offizi G, Mezzaroma I, Pandolfi F, Fiorilli M, Cassone A, Aiuti F (1995) CD8$^+$ T lymphocytes provide helper activity for IgE synthesis in human immunodeficiency virus-infected patients with Hyper-IgE. J Exp Med 181:423

119. Paganin C, Frank I, Trinchieri G (1995) Priming for high interferon-gamma production induced by interleukin-12 in both CD4$^+$ and CD8$^+$ T cell clones from HIV-infected patients. J Clin Invest 96:1677

120. Palacio J, Souberbielle BE, Shattock RJ, Robinson G, Manyonda I, Griffin GE (1994) In vitro HIV-1 infection of human cervical tissue. Res Virol 145:155

121. Pandolfi F, Oliva A, Sacco G, Polidori V, Liberatore D, Mezzaroma I, Kurnick JT, Aiuti F (1993) Fibroblast-derived factors preserve viability in vitro of mononuclear cells isolated from subjects with HIV-1 infection. J Acquir Immune Defic Syndr 7:323

122. Paxton WA, Martin SR, Tse D, O'Brien TR, Skurnick J, Vandevanter NL, Padian N, Braun JF, Kotler DP, Wolinsky SM, Koup RA (1996) Relative resistance to HIV-1 infection of CD4 lymphocytes from persons who remain uninfected despite multiple high-risk sexual exposures. Nature Med 2:412

123. Purvis SF, Jacobberger JW, Sramkoski RM, Patki AH, Lederman MM (1995) HIV type 1 Tat protein induces apoptosis and death in Jurkat cells. AIDS Res Hum Retroviruses 11:443

124. Razvi ES, Welsh RM (1993) Programmed cell death of T lymphocytes during acute viral infection: a mechanism for virus-induced immune deficiency. J Virol 67:5754

125. Richman DD, Bozzette SA (1994) The impact of the syncytium- inducing phenotype of human immunodeficiency virus on disease progression. J Infect Dis 169:968

126. Roos MTL, Miedema F, Koot M, Tersmette M, Schaasberg WP, Coutinho RA, Schellekens PTA (1995) T cell function in vitro is an independent progression marker for AIDS in human immunodeficiency virus (HIV)-infected asymptomatic individuals. J Infect Dis 171:531

127. Saag MS, Hahn BH, Gibbons J, Li Y, Parks ES, Parks WP, Shaw GM (1988) Extensive variation of human immunodeficiency virus type I in vivo. Nature 334:440

128. Salazar-Gonzalez JF, Moody DJ, Giorgi JV, Martinez-Maza O, Mitsuyasu RT, Fahey JL (1985) Reduced ecto-5'-nucleotidase activity and enhanced OKT 10 and HLA-DR expression on CD8 lymphocytes in the aquired immune deficiency syndrome: evidence of CD8 cell immaturity. J Immunol 135:1778

129. Salk J, Bretcher PA, Salk PL, Clerici M, Shearer GM (1993) A strategy for prophylactic vaccination against HIV. Science 260:1270

130. Salmon M, Pilling D, Borthwick NJ, Viner N, Janossy G, Bacon PA, Akbar AN (1994) The progressive differentiation of primed T cells is associated with an increasing susceptibility to apoptosis. Eur J Immunol 24:892

131. Schellekens PTA, Roos MTL, De Wolf F, Lange JMA, Miedema F (1990) Low T cell responsiveness to activation via CD3/TCR is a prognostic marker for AIDS in HIV-1 infected men. J Clin Immunol 10:121

132. Schellekens PTA, Tersmette M, Roos MTL, Keet R, De Wolf F, Coutinho RA, Miedema F (1992) Biphasic rate of CD4$^+$ cell decline during progression to AIDS correlates with HIV-1 phenotype. J Acquir Immune Defic Syndr 6:665

133. Schnittman SM, Psallidopoulos MC, Lane HC, Thompson L, Baseler M, Massari F, Fox CH, Salzman NP, Fauci AS (1989) The reservoir for HIV-1 in human peripheral blood is a T cell that maintains expression of CD4. Science 245:305

134. Schuitemaker H, Kootstra NA, De Goede REY, De Wolf F, Miedema F, Tersmette M (1991) Monocytotropic human immunodeficiency virus 1 (HIV-1) variants detectable in all stages of HIV infection lack T cell line tropism and syncytium-inducing ability in primary T cell culture. J Virol 65:356

135. Schuitemaker H, Koot M, Kootstra NA, Dercksen MW, De Goede REY, Van Steenwijk RP, Lange JMA, Eeftink Schattenkerk JKM, Miedema F, Tersmette M (1992) Biological phenotype of human immunodeficiency virus type 1 clones at different stages of infection: progression of disease is associated with a shift from monocytotropic to T cell-tropic virus populations. J Virol 66:1354

136. Schuitemaker H, Meyaard L, Kootstra NA, Otto SA, Dubbes R, Tersmette M, Heeney JL, Miedema F (1993) Lack of T cell dysfunction and programmed cell death in human immunodeficiency type-1 infected chimpanzees correlates with absence of monocytotropic variants. J Infect Dis 168:1140

137. Seder RA, Grabstein KH, Berzofsky JA, McDyer JF (1995) Cytokine interactions in human immunodeficiency virus-infected individuals: Roles of interleukin (IL)-2, IL-12 and IL-15. J Exp Med 182:1067

138. Shearer GM, Bernstein DC, Tung KSK, Via CS, Redfield R, Salahuddin SZ, Gallo RC (1986) A model for the selective loss of major histocompatibility complex self-restricted T cell immune responses during the development of acquired immune deficiency syndrome (AIDS). J Immunol 137:2514

139. Sheppard HW, Lang W, Ascher MS, Vittinghoff E, Winkelstein W (1993) The characterization of non-progressors: long-term HIV-1 infection with stable CD4$^+$ T cell levels. J Acquir Immune Defic Syndr 7:1159

140. Staal FJT, Ela SW, Roederer M, Anderson MT, Herzenberg LA (1992) Gluthatione deficiency and human immunodeficiency virus infection. Lancet 339:909

141. Stites DP, Moss AR, Bacchetti P, Osmond D, McHugh TM, Wang YJ, Hebert S, Colfer B (1989) Lymphocyte subset analysis to predict progression to AIDS in a cohort of homosexual men in San Francisco. Clin Immunol Immunopathol 52:96

142. Tamaru Y, Miyawaki T, Iwai K, Tsuji T, Nibu R, Yachie A, Koizumi S, Taniguchi N (1993) Absence of bcl-2 expression by acivated CD45RO$^+$ T lymphocytes in acute infectious mononucleosis supporting their susceptibility to programmed cell death. Blood 82:521

143. Teppler H, Kaplan G, Smith K, Cameron P, Montana A, Meyn P, Cohn Z (1993) Efficacy of low doses of the polyethylene glycol derivative of interleukin-2 in modulating the immune response of patients with human immunodeficiency virus type 1 infection. J Infect Dis 167:291

144. Teppler H, Kaplan G, Smith KA, Montana AL, Meyn P, Cohn ZA (1993) Prolonged immunostimulatory effect of low-dose polyethylene glycol interleukin 2 in patients with human immunodeficiency virus type 1 infection. J Exp Med 177:483

145. Terai C, Kornbluth RS, Pauza CD, Richman DD, Carson DA (1991) Apoptosis as a mechanism of cell death in cultured T lymphoblasts acutely infected with HIV-1. J Clin Invest 87:1710

146. Tersmette M, De Goede REY, Al BJM, Winkel IN, Gruters RA, Cuypers HTM, Huisman HG, Miedema F (1988) Differential syncytium-inducing capacity of human immunodeficiency virus isolates: frequent detection of syncytium-inducing isolates in patients with acquired immunodeficiency syndrome (AIDS) and AIDS-related complex. J Virol 62:2026

147. Tersmette M, Lange JMA, De Goede REY, De Wolf F, Eeftink Schattenkerk JKM, Schellekens PThA, Coutinho RA, Huisman JG, Goudsmit J, Miedema F (1989) Association between biological properties of human immunodeficiency virus variants and risk for AIDS and AIDS mortality. Lancet I:983

148. Tindall B, Cooper DA (1991) Primary HIV infection: host responses and intervention strategies. J Acquir Immune Defic Syndr 5:1

149. Uehara T, Miyawaki T, Ohta K, Tamaru Y, Yokoi T, Nakamura S, Taniguchi N (1992) Apoptotic cell death of primed CD45RO$^+$ T lymphocytes in Epstein-Barr virus induced infectious mononucleosis. Blood 80:452

150. Van 't Wout AB, Kootstra NA, Mulder-Kampinga GA, Albrecht MA, Scherpbier HJ, Veenstra J, Boer K, Coutinho RA, Miedema F, Schuitemaker H (1994) Macrophage-tropic variants initiate human immunodeficiency virus type 1 infection after sexual, parenteral and vertical transmission. J Clin Invest 94:2060

151. Van den Berg AP, Meyaard L, Otto SA, Van Son WJ, Klompmaker IJ, Mesander G, De Leij LHFM, Miedema F, The TH (1995) Cytomegalovirus infection associated with a decreased proliferative capacity and increased rate of apoptosis of peripheral blood lymphocytes. Transplant Proc 27:936

152. Von Briesen H, Becker WB, Henco K, Helm EB, Gelderblom HR, Brede HD, Rubsamen-Waigmann H (1987) Isolation frequency and growth properties of HIV variants: multiple simultaneous variants in a patient demonstrated by molecular cloning. J Med Virol 23:51

153. Vyakarnam A, Matear P, Meager A, Kelly G, Stanley B, Weller I, Beverley P (1991) Altered production of tumour necrosis factors alpha and beta and interferon gamma by HIV-infected individuals. Clin Exp Immunol 84:109

154. Walker CM, Levy JA (1989) A diffusible lymphokine produced by CD8$^+$ T lymphocytes suppresses HIV replication. Immunology 66:628

155. Walker CM, Erickson AL, Hsueh FC, Levy JP (1991) Inhibition of human immunodeficiency virus replication in acutely infected CD4+ cells by CD8+ cells involves a noncytotoxic mechanism. J Virol 65:5921

156. Walker CM, Thomson-Honnebier GA, Hsueh FC, Erickson AL, Pan LZ, Levy JA (1991) CD8+ T cells from HIV-1 infected individuals inhibit acute infection by human and primate immunodeficiency viruses. Cell Immunol 137:420

157. Wang R, Murphy KM, Loh DY, Weaver C, Russell JH (1993) Differential activation of antigen-stimulated suicide and cytokine production pathways in CD4+ T cells is regulated by the antigen-presenting cell. J Immunol 150:3832

158. Wei X, Ghosh SK, Taylor ME, Johnson VA, Emini EA, Deutsch P, Lifson JD, Bonhoeffer S, Nowak MA, Hahn BH, Saag MS, Shaw GM (1995) Viral dynamics in human immunodeficiency virus type1 infection. Nature 373:117

159. Wesselborg S, Janssen O, Kabelitz D (1993) Induction of activation-driven death (apoptosis) in activated but not resting peripheral blood T cells. J Immunol 150:4338

160. Westendorp MO, Frank R, Ochsenbauer C, Stricker K, Dhein J, Walczak H, Debatin K-M, Krammer PH (1995) Sensitization to CD95-mediated apoptosis by HIV-1 Tat and gp120. Nature 375:497

161. Wiviott LD, Walker CM, Levy JA (1990) CD8+ lymphocytes suppress HIV production by autologous CD4+ cells without eliminating the infected cells. Cell Immunol 128:628

162. Wood R, Montoya JG, Kundu SK, Schwartz DH, Merigan TC (1993) Safety and efficacy of polyethylene glycol-modified interleukin-2 and zidovudine in human immunodeficiency virus type 1 infection: a phase I/II study. J Infect Dis 167:519

163. Yssel H, De Waal Malefyt R, Roncarolo MG, Abrams JS, Lahesmaa R, Spits H, De Vries JE (1992) IL-10 is produced by subsets of human CD4+ T cell clones and peripheral blood T cells. J Immunol 149:2378

164. Yssel H, Fasler S, De Vries JE, De Waal Malefyt R (1994) IL-12 transiently induces IFN-gamma transcription and protein synthesis in human CD4+ allergen-specific Th2 T cell clones. Int Immunol 6:1091

165. Zauli G, Vitale M, Re MC, Furlini G, Zamai L, Falcieri E, Gibellini D, Visani G, Davis BR, Capitani S, La Placa M (1994) In vitro exposure to human immunodeficiency virus type 1 induces apoptotic cell death of the factor-dependent TF-1 hematopoietic cell line. Blood 83:167

166. Zhang M, Gong J, Iyer DV, Jones BE, Modlin RL, Barnes PF (1994) T cell cytokine responses in persons with tuberculosis and human immunodeficiency virus infection. J Clin Invest 94:2435

167. Zinkernagel RM, Hengartner H (1994) T cell mediated immunopathology versus direct cytolysis by virus: implications for HIV and AIDS. Immunol Today 15:262

Studies on lymphoid tissue from HIV-infected individuals: implications for the design of therapeutic strategies

Oren J. Cohen, Giuseppe Pantaleo, Gordon K. Lam, Anthony S. Fauci

Laboratory of Immunoregulation, National Institute of Allergy and Infectious Diseases, National Institutes of Health, 10 Center Drive MSC 1876, Building 10, Room 11B13, Bethesda, MD 20892–1876, USA

Summary. Lymphoid tissue is a major reservoir of human immunodeficiency virus (HIV) infection in vivo. In addition, the lymphoid microenvironment provides a replicative advantage to the virus in that it provides a milieu of activated target cells that allows for efficient virus spread. The process of mobilization and activation of immune competent cells directed against the virus paradoxically contributes to the propagation of virus replication. Disruption of the lymphoid microenvironment during the progression of HIV disease is a poorly understood process, which may be of considerable importance pathogenically. Studies of lymph node biopsy samples taken 8 weeks apart from individuals who did not undergo any change in their therapeutic regimen (i.e., patients who either remained untreated or remained on their ongoing nucleoside analogue reverse transcriptase inhibitor monotherapy regimen) revealed little change in histopathology or viral load over the 8-week period. These results with successive lymph node biopsy samples taken from different sites indicate that an isolated lymph node biopsy accurately reflects the pathologic process associated with HIV infection and that this process diffusely involves the lymphoid system. Treatment with reverse transcriptase inhibitor monotherapy of patients in relatively early stage HIV disease had no detectable impact on the viral load in lymphoid tissue, suggesting the need to investigate more potent antiretroviral regimens during this stage of disease. Among patients with moderately advanced HIV disease, switching to combination therapy from a monotherapy regimen resulted in decreased viral replication in lymph nodes; this effect was associated with decreases in plasma viremia. Despite the fact that measures of viral replication decreased significantly, the net frequency of HIV-infected cells in peripheral blood and lymph nodes remained unchanged. Potent antiretroviral drug combinations may be capable of profound and long-term down-regulation of plasma viremia. It will be essential to monitor the status of viral trapping, viral burden, and viral replication within lymphoid tissue during treatment with such drugs to determine accurately their true potential for impact on these key features of HIV pathogenesis.

Correspondence to: O.J. Cohen

HIV within the microenvironment of lymphoid tissue

During the generally prolonged period of asymptomatic HIV infection, virologic parameters such as p24 antigenemia and titers of infectious virus in plasma and peripheral blood mononuclear cells (PBMC) are relatively low. These low levels of viral load are inconsistent with the progressive decline of CD4$^+$ T lymphocyte numbers and immune dysfunction which characterize this period of infection [1]. Studies employing sensitive polymerase chain reaction (PCR) technology have demonstrated that plasma viremia is detectable throughout the entire course of HIV infection, explaining in part the apparent discrepancy between the relatively low frequency of HIV-infected cells in peripheral blood and the progressive decline in CD4$^+$ T cell numbers and immune function [2, 3]. Furthermore, a critical study which compared viral burden (i.e., the frequency of cells harboring HIV DNA) and viral replication in mononuclear cells obtained from peripheral blood and lymph nodes of the same individuals demonstrated that viral burden in lymph nodes exceeds that in peripheral blood by 5- to 10-fold; furthermore, viral replication in lymph nodes is generally 10- to 100-fold greater than that in PBMC [4, 5]. Another study utilized in situ PCR to demonstrate that up to 25% of CD4$^+$ T lymphocytes present in lymph node germinal centers harbor HIV DNA, further emphasizing the role of lymphoid tissue as a critical reservoir for HIV in vivo [6]. More recent studies have shown that plasma viremia is in a continuous state of rapid high-level turnover ($> 10^9$ virions produced daily) and that virions in plasma most likely derive from viral replication in lymphoid tissue [7–9].

The anatomical and immunological events which occur in peripheral lymphoid tissue following introduction of antigen have been recently reviewed [10]. Immature tissue dendritic cells efficiently take up antigens and migrate to lymph nodes via the afferent lymphatics. In the paracortical areas, antigen-laden dendritic cells stimulate naive T cells by virtue of T cell receptor–antigen as well as CD28–B7 interactions. Migration of activated T cells into follicles stimulates B cell proliferation, antibody production and isotype switching, and germinal center formation via CD40 ligand–CD40 interaction as well as by elaboration of lymphokines. Follicular dendritic cells (FDC) bind antigen-antibody complexes in germinal centers and serve to stimulate affinity maturation of the B cell response.

In the earliest phases of primary infection with HIV, viral RNA is detected in association with large numbers of productively infected T cells in the paracortical regions of lymph nodes [11]. High levels of plasma viremia reflect unimpeded viral replication within lymphoid tissue. Generation of cellular and humoral immune responses against HIV are responsible for the subsequent patterns of viral trapping within lymph node germinal centers and of individual cells expressing HIV RNA in the paracortical areas [11]. Cellular immune responses are likely responsible for the substantial elimination (i.e., one to two orders of magnitude) of productively infected T cells from the paracortical regions of lymph nodes, a process which curtails the supply of virions to the plasma compartment [12, 13]. Production of anti-HIV antibodies results in formation of immune complexes which are then cleared from the circulation. Concurrent expansion of the FDC network within hyperplastic lymphoid follicles is an efficient mechanism for viral trapping via interactions between antibody and complement-coated virions and FDC receptor molecules for complement (i.e., C3b and C3d on the surface of FDC) [14, 15]. Thus, during the chronic phase of infection with HIV, most viral RNA is detected as extracellular virions closely

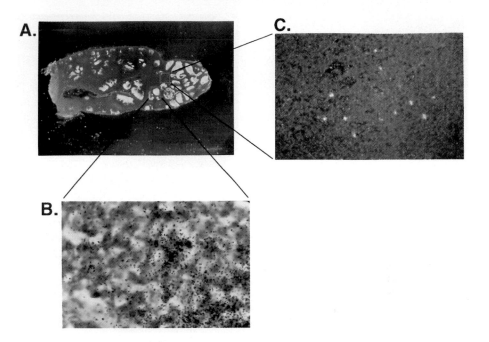

Fig. 1A–C. The microenvironment of interactions between lymph nodes and HIV. **A** In situ hybridization for HIV RNA shown by dark field microscopy. Accumulation of white grains, corresponding to HIV RNA, is seen predominantly within germinal centers. **B** CD21 immunostaining (*red*) highlights the processes of follicular dendritic cells (FDC) within germinal centers, while HIV RNA detected by in situ hybridization appears as black grains by light field microscopy. The pattern of HIV RNA deposition is nearly superimposable with that of the FDC processes. **C** In situ hybridization for HIV RNA viewed by dark field microscopy in the paracortical region. Individual lymphocytes which are productively infected and expressing HIV RNA are seen. **A** ×13; **B, C** ×1000

associated with the FDC network (Fig. 1). The presence of productively infected T cells is detected to a greater or lesser extent, likely dependent on the efficiency of cellular immune control of viral replication (Fig. 1).

As HIV disease progresses, there is a shift in the lymphoid histopathologic pattern from follicular hyperplasia to follicular involution [16, 17]. This shift in histopathology is associated with important changes in viral distribution. Disruption of the FDC network is characteristic during the transition from follicular hyperplasia to involution. This leads to a decrease in the efficiency of viral trapping in germinal centers (Fig. 2), which contributes together with the acceleration in virus replication to an increase in plasma viremia [5, 11]. Sequestration of infected cells within lymphoid tissue also becomes less efficient during follicular involution. Thus, changes in the levels of viral burden and replication in lymph nodes and peripheral blood may in part reflect redistribution of viral load between these two compartments. Distribution of viral load between the lymph node and peripheral blood compartments is determined by the integrity of the FDC network [9, 18]; an intact FDC network serves as a filter between the compartments, whereas a disrupted network will allow more direct communication. This point is illustrated by a patient who underwent two lymph node biopsies, separated by 8 weeks, following a switch from a monotherapy regimen to combination nucleoside analogue reverse transcriptase inhibitor (RTI) therapy (Fig. 3).

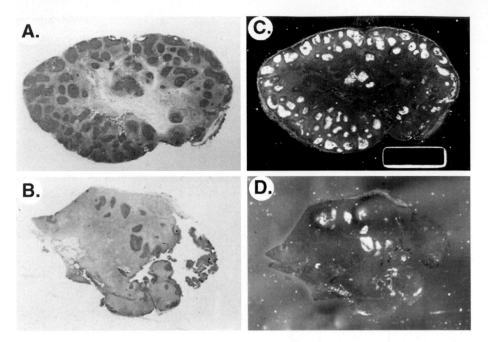

Fig. 2A–D. Disruption of the FDC network leads to decreased viral trapping in lymph nodes. **A, C** A lymph node from a patient with a CD4$^+$ T cell count of 647 cells/μl is shown. **B, D** A lymph node from a patient with more advanced disease with a CD4$^+$ T cell count of 389 cells/μl is shown. **A, B** CD21 immunostain; **C, D** in situ hybridization for HIV RNA after protease digestion

Levels of viral replication in the lymph nodes unexpectedly increased 20-fold over the 8 week period; however, no change was detected in plasma viremia. Histopathologic examination of the lymph node revealed follicular hyperplasia and extensive trapping of virions in germinal centers, suggesting that by virtue of efficient viral trapping capacity, an intact FDC network may inhibit release of newly formed virions from lymph nodes to the plasma compartment [9].

In the advanced stage of HIV disease there is almost total dissolution of lymphoid architecture. Destruction of lymphoid tissue certainly is a major factor in the severe immune dysfunction and loss of ability to inhibit viral replication. The ability to mount immune responses against new antigens and the ability to maintain memory responses is severely impaired in the absence of intact lymphoid tissue architecture. Included among these defective immune responses are those directed against HIV itself, resulting in increased cell-associated viral RNA in the paracortical regions of lymph nodes. Thus, during progression of HIV disease there is a reversal in the predominant forms of virus in the lymph nodes. There is progressive diminution of the extracellular form (i.e., trapped virus) and an increase in cell-associated virus (i.e., cells expressing HIV) [5, 11]. Follicular involution, fibrosis, frank lymphocyte depletion, and fatty infiltration herald complete loss of functional lymphoid tissue, contributing to the dramatically enhanced susceptibility of the patient to opportunistic infections.

A central dilemma in understanding the pathogenesis of HIV infection is the failure of the immune system of the host to completely eliminate the virus. The ability of HIV to subvert the immune system to its own replicative advantage is surely

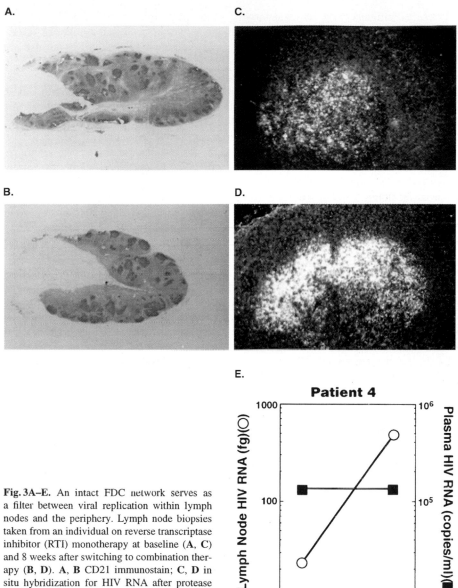

Fig. 3A–E. An intact FDC network serves as a filter between viral replication within lymph nodes and the periphery. Lymph node biopsies taken from an individual on reverse transcriptase inhibitor (RTI) monotherapy at baseline (**A, C**) and 8 weeks after switching to combination therapy (**B, D**). **A, B** CD21 immunostain; **C, D** in situ hybridization for HIV RNA after protease digestion. The intact FDC network which efficiently traps virus may explain the stable levels of plasma viremia despite a significant increase in HIV replication in lymph node (**E**)

an important pathogenic mechanism. The microenvironment of lymphoid tissue is ideally suited to maintain a high degree of immune activation. Close contact between immune effector cells and the high levels of pro-inflammatory cytokines [e.g., tumor necrosis factor (TNF)-α, interleukin (IL)-1β, and IL-6] produced in lymph nodes that harbor efficiently trapped, potentially infectious virions [19] favor viral replication in several ways. Activated CD4$^+$ T lymphocytes migrating through lymphoid tissue in response to antigens serve as ideal targets for de novo infection with HIV [20–23]. Pro-inflammatory cytokines, found in abundance within activated lymphoid tissue, are potent inducers of HIV replication in latently infected cells [24–28] and also are able to increase the pool of activated cells that are susceptible to HIV infection [20, 24, 25, 29]. Sequestration of HIV-infected cells within lymphoid tissue may also contribute to the dichotomy in viral load between lymph node and peripheral blood. This sequestration may result from defective egress of cells due to histopathologic abnormalities and cytokine imbalances [30].

Disruption of the lymphoid microenvironment during the course of HIV infection remains an enigmatic process with substantial implications for the design of therapeutic strategies. Dissolution of the FDC network may result from a number of direct or indirect HIV- mediated mechanisms. Productive infection of FDC by HIV is a potential mechanism for which there is some support, particularly in the late stages of HIV infection ([31] and G Pantaleo and AS Fauci, unpublished observations); however, the majority of data suggest that productive infection of FDC is rare during the intermediate stage of HIV disease when dissolution of the FDC network begins [32]. Direct toxicity of viral gene products may contribute to loss of integrity of the FDC network. Gp120 and/or tat have been shown to be capable of disrupting normal intracellular signalling [33, 34] as well as inducing apoptosis [35–37]. Although these effects have been studied largely in CD4$^+$ T cells, little is known regarding the normal physiology of FDC and their interactions with HIV proteins. Tat has been shown to down-regulate MHC class 1 expression [38], which may interfere with normal cell-cell interactions in the lymphoid microenvironment. Depletion of CD4$^+$ T cells during the course of HIV disease could lead to withdrawal of a trophic factor necessary for FDC survival. Induction by HIV of tissue-damaging gene products may contribute to disruption of the FDC network over time; candidate mediators include nitric oxide [39–41] and matrix metalloproteinases such as MMP-9 [42, 43]. An "innocent bystander" phenomenon is also a possibility, wherein cells (e.g., CD8$^+$ T cells, macrophages) infiltrating into hyperplastic lymph nodes elaborate substances (e.g., TNF-α) that may be toxic at high sustained concentrations.

Lymph node pathology reflects a systemic process throughout lymphoid tissue

The effects of antiretroviral therapy on virologic and histopathologic parameters in lymphoid tissue were studied by performing lymph node biopsies at baseline and after 8 weeks. Initiation of RTI monotherapy or conversion of monotherapy to combination therapy was studied [9, 44]. The baseline mean CD4$^+$ T cell count in the previously untreated group was 659 cells/μl, whereas in the group already receiving RTI monotherapy representing patients with more advanced HIV disease the baseline mean CD4$^+$ T cell count was 406 cells/μl. The control groups (i.e., those who remained untreated and those who remained on their ongoing regimen of RTI monotherapy) provided important data regarding the reliability of any given lymph node biopsy in reflecting the pathologic process diffusely present in lymphoid tissue. The data indicated that virologic and immunologic parameters of HIV infection in lymphoid tissue are part of a systemic process, and that a single lymph node is representative of that process [9, 44].

Histopathologic staging was performed according to the relative degrees of follicular hyperplasia and follicular involution. The pattern of HIV-related histologic abnormalities remained constant in each patient over the 8-week study. Thus, when follicular hyperplasia was the dominant pattern seen in the baseline lymph node, it tended to also be the dominant pattern in the week 8 lymph node, regardless of treatment. Among control patients (i.e., those who did not undergo any change in therapy), 81% of week 8 nodes were classified at the identical stage as their baseline counterparts (Fig. 4) [44].

In situ hybridization for HIV RNA also revealed no change in the distribution pattern of viral RNA within lymph nodes (Fig. 4); consistent with previous studies, trapped virus was detected in the FDC network within germinal centers [5, 15, 16, 45, 46]. Morphometric analysis of the percentage of lymph node area occupied by CD21 immunostain (i.e., relative germinal center area) revealed no significant change in relative germinal center area among those patients who remained untreated (22.9% at baseline; 27.1% at week 8) as well as among those patients who remained on their ongoing regimen of RTI monotherapy (17.0% at baseline; 19.5% at week 8). The same pattern was seen when morphometric analysis of the percentage of lymph node area occupied by HIV RNA signal was performed. The relative HIV area was 9.0% at baseline and 10.1% at week 8 among those patients who remained untreated and 6.0% at baseline and 7.3% at week 8 among those patients who remained on RTI monotherapy (Fig. 5).

The frequency of HIV-infected cells (viral burden) measured by PCR remained constant over the 8 week period in lymph node mononuclear cells (MC) from both control groups (i.e., those who remained untreated and those who remained on RTI monotherapy). In those patients who remained untreated, mean viral burden per 10^6 lymph node MC was 2722 HIV DNA copies at baseline and 2441 copies at week 8 (Table 1). Among patients who remained on RTI monotherapy, mean viral burden per 10^6 lymph node MC was 4233 at baseline and 4876 at week 8 (Table 2). There were also no significant changes in levels of virus replication (i.e., HIV RNA levels measured by RT-PCR) in lymph node MC in either group which did not undergo a change in therapy. In those who remained untreated, HIV RNA levels (per 1.5 μg total cellular RNA) in lymph node MC were 131 fg and 302 fg at baseline and week 8 respectively (Table 1), while in those who remained on RTI monotherapy the corresponding values were 137 fg and 107 fg (Table 2).

Studies involving baseline and week 8 lymph node biopsies from each patient who either remained untreated or remained on an ongoing regimen of RTI monotherapy allowed for an assessment of possible sampling error. The remarkable consistency between baseline and week 8 with regard to histopathologic and virologic findings in biopsy samples of each patient indicate that a lymph node biopsy is a reliable indicator of the status of the lymphoid system as a whole during the course of HIV disease [9, 44, 47].

Treatment of early stage HIV disease with RTI monotherapy

Initiation of RTI monotherapy in patients with fewer than 500 CD4$^+$ T cells/μl of peripheral blood increases CD4$^+$ T cell counts and has been shown to decrease parameters of viral replication (p24 antigenemia and plasma viremia), and to delay progression to AIDS [48–52]. The rationale for initiation of treatment at earlier stages of disease was strengthened by studies which showed significant and persistent HIV replication even during the early, clinically latent period of HIV disease [3, 5]. Ini-

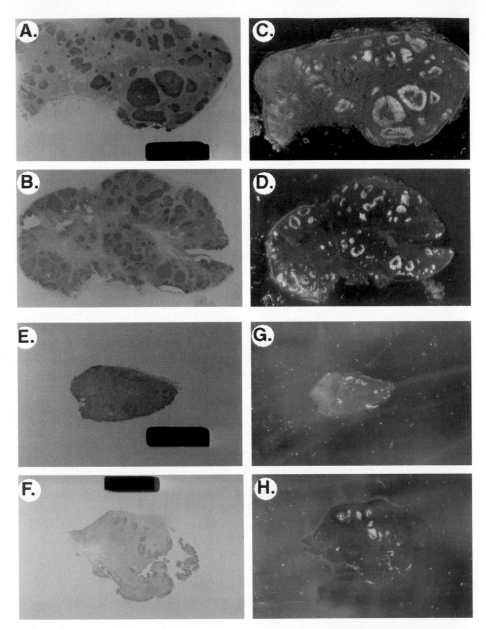

Fig. 4A–H. Lymph node biopsy samples from the same individuals taken 8 weeks apart without any change in therapy show consistency in histopathologic abnormalities. **A** and **B**, **E** and **F** CD21 immunostain showing a similar degree of follicular hyperplasia in the lymph nodes of two patients when each week 8 biopsy (**B**, **F**) is compared with baseline (**A**, **E**). **C** and **D**, **G** and **H** In situ hybridization for HIV RNA after protease digestion showing a similar degree of viral trapping in germinal centers of the same two patients when each week 8 biopsy (**D**, **H**) is compared with baseline (**C**, **G**)

tiation of antiretroviral therapy in the early stages of HIV disease seems to increase CD4$^+$ T cell counts; however, clinical benefits have been difficult to demonstrate [53–

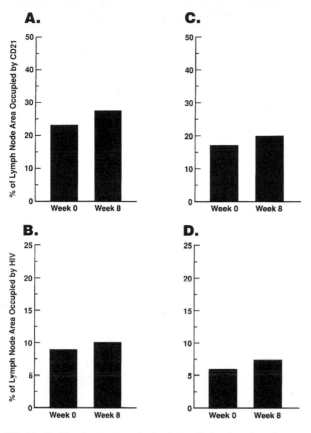

Fig. 5A–D. Morphometric analysis of the relative lymph node area occupied by CD21 immunostain and by HIV RNA shows consistency in the degree of follicular hyperplasia and viral trapping, respectively. Morphometric analysis of CD21 immunostain and HIV RNA in lymph nodes of patients who remained untreated (**A** and **B**) and who remained on RTI monotherapy (**C** and **D**)

55]. One caveat in the interpretation of such studies is the question of how reliable are surrogate markers of HIV disease, such as CD4+ T cell counts [56]. Another major caveat regarding the interpretation of changes in surrogate markers in peripheral blood following initiation of antiretroviral therapy is the possibility that the peripheral blood compartment may not be an accurate indicator of pathogenic processes within lymphoid tissue, which is considered to be the major reservoir of HIV and the primary site of HIV replication [4–6, 15, 16, 25, 45, 46, 57, 58]. It was, therefore, important to conduct a study of initiation of antiretroviral therapy that included analysis of lymph node biopsy samples as well as peripheral blood markers.

Antiretroviral-naive, HIV+ patients with a baseline mean CD4+ T cell count of 659 cells/μl were studied with lymph node and peripheral blood sampling at baseline and again after 8 weeks of either remaining untreated or initiating RTI monotherapy [44]. In the control group (i.e., those who remained untreated), no change was seen in CD4+ T cell counts, viral burden in PBMC, or plasma viremia over the 8 week study period (Table 1). As noted above, all histopathologic and virologic parameters measured in lymph nodes also remained constant in the control group (Table 1). Among patients who initiated RTI monotherapy, the mean CD4+ T cell count increased from 655

Table 1. The effect of reverse transcriptase inhibitor (RTI) monotherapy in early stage HIV disease on immunologic and virologic parameters in peripheral blood and lymph nodes

	Group:			
	Untreated: remained untreated		Untreated: initiated RTI	
	Week 0	Week 8	Week 0	Week 8
CD4+ T cells/μl	664	658	655	804
Viral burden PBMC[a]	688	661	894	848
Plasma viremia[b]	180678	74479	24250	6593
Viral burden LNMC[a]	2722	2441	3196	3336
Viral replication LNMC[c]	131	302	173	283
CD21% in lymph node[d]	22.9	27.1	24.0	21.5
HIV% in lymph node[e]	9.0	10.1	13.8	10.9

PBMC, Peripheral blood mononuclear cells; LNMC, lymph node mononuclear cells

[a] Viral burden expressed as HIV DNA copies/10^6 mononuclear cells

[b] Plasma viremia expressed as HIV RNA copies/ml plasma

[c] Viral replication expressed as fg equivalents of HIV RNA/1.5 μg total cellular RNA

[d] Percentage of lymph nodal area occupied by CD21 stain (i.e., relative degree of follicular hyperplasia) determined by immunocytochemistry and morphometric analysis

[e] percentage of lymph nodal area occupied by HIV RNA (i.e., relative degree of viral trapping in germinal centers) determined by in situ hybridization and morphometric analysis

cells/μl at baseline to 804 cells/μl at week 8 (Table 1); however, this change was not statistically significant. Viral burden in PBMC remained unchanged over the 8 week study, as did plasma viremia (Table 1). The effects of RTI monotherapy on variables measured in lymphoid tissue also did not change during the study. Overall, there were no acute changes in patterns of histopathology (i.e., the relative degrees of follicular hyperplasia and involution) or in patterns of viral trapping within germinal centers. There were no detectable changes seen in viral burden and levels of virus replication in lymph node MC (Table 1).

The lack of effect of RTI monotherapy on viral load in peripheral blood and lymph nodes in this group of patients in early stage HIV disease was due neither to the baseline prevalence of resistant virus (present in only 1 out of the 16 patients) nor to the development of resistant virus over the 8 week period (which did not occur in a single case) [44]. Measurement of drug levels in lymph node MC further suggested that the negative results could not be explained by lack of penetration of drug into lymphoid tissue [44]. It is possible that the relatively small sample size of the study and/or the limits of sensitivity of the assays used in the study precluded detection of small but real changes in viral load. Future studies of potent combination antiretroviral regimens should yield important information regarding the possibility of decreasing viral load from a relatively low level in the early stages of HIV disease; whether or not the natural history of HIV disease can be altered by such an intervention remains an open question.

Table 2. The effect of combination antiretroviral therapy in moderately advanced stage HIV disease on immunologic and virologic parameters in peripheral blood and lymph nodes

| | Group: | | | |
| | Monotherapy: remained on monotherapy | | Monotherapy: switch to combination | |
	week 0	week 8	week 0	week 8
CD4+ T cells/μl	413	408	394	436
Viral burden PBMC[a]	1338	1572	1539	1187
Plasma viremia[b]	40 128	86 360	179 927	46730*
Viral burden LNMC[a]	4233	4876	4438	3799
Viral replication LNMC[c]	137	107	486	164
CD21% in lymph node[d]	17.0	19.5	15.9	16.3
HIV% in lymph node[e]	6.0	7.3	7.2	7.1

[a] Viral burden expressed as HIV DNA copies/10^6 mononuclear cells
[b] Plasma viremia expressed as HIV RNA copies/ml plasma
[c] Viral replication expressed as fg equivalents of HIV RNA/1.5 μg total cellular RNA
[d] Percentage of lymph nodal area occupied by CD21 stain (i.e., relative degree of follicular hyperplasia) determined by immunocytochemistry and morphometric analysis
[e] Percentage of lymph nodal area occupied by HIV RNA (i.e., relative degree of viral trapping in germinal centers) determined by in situ hybridization and morphometric analysis
* $P < 0.05$

Treatment of moderately advanced HIV disease with combination antiretroviral therapy

Parallel analysis of changes in viral load in lymph nodes and peripheral blood after conversion of RTI monotherapy to combination therapy represented an ideal opportunity to determine the lymphoid tissue correlates of expected decreases in plasma viremia. Patients receiving a regimen of RTI monotherapy underwent lymph node biopsy and peripheral blood sampling at baseline and after 8 weeks of either remaining on monotherapy or receiving an additional antiretroviral agent [9]. The baseline mean CD4+ T cell count for the group was 406 cells/μl. Among patients who remained on monotherapy, there were no changes in peripheral blood markers (CD4+ T cell counts, viral burden in PBMC, and plasma viremia) or lymph node markers (viral burden and viral replication in lymph node MC; Table 2). Among those who switched to the combination therapy regimen, most experienced decreases in plasma viremia which paralleled decreases in virus replication in lymph node MC [9] (Fig. 6); this correlation has recently been confirmed in a study of zidovudine, didanosine, and lamivudine therapy during which serial lymph node biopsy and plasma specimens were obtained [59]. In spite of substantial decreases in virus replication in lymph node MC and in plasma viremia, viral burden in PBMC and lymph node MC remained unchanged (Table 2).

Plasma viremia is an important prognostic marker during the course of HIV infection. High levels of plasma viremia have negative prognostic significance in their own right [60], and decreases in plasma viremia during antiretroviral therapy have been shown to predict clinical efficacy [61]. The relationship between plasma viremia

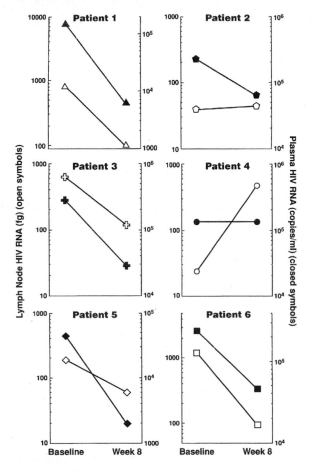

Fig. 6. Decreases in viral replication in lymph nodes are paralleled by decreases in plasma viremia for four of six patients who switched to combination therapy from a monotherapy regimen (patients 1, 3, 5, and 6). *Open symbols* indicate HIV RNA in lymph node mononuclear cells; *solid symbols* indicate plasma viremia (adapted from [9])

and viral load in lymph node compartments is complex. At steady state there does not appear to be a correlation between absolute levels of plasma viremia and levels of virus replication in lymphoid tissue ([62] and O Cohen, G Pantaleo, and AS Fauci; unpublished observations); however, decreases in plasma viremia on therapy tend to correlate with decreases in levels of virus replication in lymphoid tissue. This apparent paradox may be due to the relative virus-trapping capacity of the FDC network within lymph nodes. Again, an intact FDC network may serve as a filter between high levels of virus replication in lymphoid tissue and relatively low levels of plasma viremia. The fact that decreases in levels of virus replication in lymphoid tissue are mirrored by decreases in plasma viremia does, however, indicate that at least a substantial fraction of plasma viremia is dependent upon virus replication in lymphoid tissue [9].

Another interesting finding was that during combination antiretroviral therapy, the frequency of HIV-infected cells (i.e., viral burden) remained essentially unchanged despite modest decreases in levels of virus replication. Nucleoside analogues, by virtue of their inhibition of RT, should prevent infection of target cells and should have no effect on cells which have already been infected. Therefore, the results are consistent with reports that much of the viral replication at any given point in time emanates from a relatively small population of newly infected target cells [7–9].

Insights into HIV pathogenesis from studies on the effects of therapy on viral load in different compartments

Ongoing studies of potent combination antiretroviral regimens given to patients in the acute phase of HIV infection have shown that plasma viremia can be suppressed for prolonged periods to levels below the current limits of detectability [63–65]. Such treatment may alter the natural history of HIV disease [66]; however, it will be essential to monitor viral load in the lymphoid compartment of these patients to maximize understanding of the relationship between viral load and pathogenesis of HIV disease.

The quantitative relationship between changes in viral load in the plasma and lymphoid compartments remains an important and unanswered question. Plasma viremia is proportional to the number of productively infected cells (which are concentrated in lymphoid tissue) and the burst size of virions produced by these cells. The relative effect of different therapeutic interventions on these variables in vivo is currently unknown. It is reasonable to expect that during potent combination antiretroviral therapy with protease inhibitors and RTI, the following scenario may occur: productively infected lymphocytes die either due to direct viral effects or to immune targeting; infection of new cells is inhibited by RTI; and the burst size of infected long-lived cells (e.g., tissue macrophages) is decreased by protease inhibitors. Such a scenario is hinted at by the decay in plasma viremia during combination therapy. The decay is extremely rapid in the days following initiation of therapy, likely reflecting the death of productively infected cells and prevention of de novo infections; however, a second, slow decay (measured in weeks) in plasma viremia may be due to a decrease in viral burst size from infected tissue macrophages and the slower turnover of these cells [67].

It will be important to delineate the kinetics of the decay in plasma viremia and viral replication in lymphoid tissue during therapy. The slower decay in viral replication from cells in lymphoid tissue [9, 59] compared with the more rapid decay in plasma viremia may be due to the filtering capacity of the FDC network. In this regard, monitoring of plasma viremia during therapy must be done with the recognition that decreases in plasma viremia may overestimate the therapeutic effect of the regimen in question. As noted above (see Fig. 6, patient 4), an increase in viral replication in lymph node cells may be absorbed in situ by an intact FDC network resulting in no change in plasma viremia. Decreases in viral replication from lymph node cells will thus appear magnified when plasma viremia is measured, due to the filtering capacity of the FDC network which separates the compartments.

Because of the fact that extracellular virions trapped within the FDC network remain infectious [19], it is essential to consider this compartment in studies on the effect of therapy on viral kinetics. During therapy with antiretroviral agents of modest potency, no change in the degree of virus trapping within germinal centers was noted [9]. The new generation of potent combination antiretroviral regimens which include protease inhibitors should allow approximation of the half-life of trapped virions. The potential role of this reservoir of HIV in de novo infection of CD4$^+$ T cells trafficking through germinal centers should not be underestimated.

Summary and conclusions

Lymphoid tissue is a critical reservoir for HIV in vivo. The relationship between the lymph node microenvironment and HIV follows a well-characterized pattern over the course of disease progression. During primary HIV infection, viral RNA is detected in association with productively infected T cells in the paracortical areas. The emergence of anti-HIV cell-mediated immune responses is temporally associated with the elimination of a large percentage of these productively infected cells as well as with a significant reduction in plasma viremia which follows primary infection. The emergence of anti-HIV humoral immune responses is likely also responsible for reducing plasma viremia via formation of immune complexes (i.e., virions plus antibodies plus complement) and deposition of these complexes on the processes of FDC in germinal centers. The hallmark of disease progression in lymphoid tissue is disruption of lymphoid tissue architecture, especially with regard to the FDC network. Follicular hyperplasia gives way to follicular involution, fibrosis, and even lymphocyte depletion. Disruption of lymphoid tissue architecture is associated with loss of viral trapping capacity, which may in turn lead to increased plasma viremia due, at least in part, to redistribution of virus from the lymphoid compartment to the plasma. Plasma viremia may also increase during this period due to diminution of immunologic control over virus replication, resulting from dissolution of the lymphoid tissue microenvironment.

Attention to the role of lymphoid tissue in the pathogenesis of HIV disease should provide insights into the development of therapeutic strategies. Failure of the host immune response to completely eliminate HIV and the ability of HIV to subvert the immune response to its own replicative advantage are important considerations in this regard. Viral trapping in germinal centers and viral replication in paracortical T cells result in the mobilization of both humoral and cell-mediated immune responses. The consequent milieu of pro-inflammatory cytokines and cellular activation may stimulate HIV replication directly and also serve to increase the pool of target cells for de novo infection. Rational therapeutic interventions based on this model include not only inhibition of viral replication, but also inhibition of viral trapping in germinal centers, counter-regulation or neutralization of pro-inflammatory cytokines, and inhibition of cellular activation. Other interventions will await delineation of the mechanisms responsible for the disruption of lymphoid tissue architecture.

Studies of lymph node biopsies performed at baseline and after 8 weeks of no intervention (i.e., continuation of no therapy in a group of HIV-infected patients in early stage disease or continuation of a stable regimen of RTI monotherapy in a group of patients with moderately advanced disease) demonstrated remarkable consistency in histopathologic and virologic parameters over this relatively short interval. These results indicate that parameters examined in a single lymph node are quite representative of a pathologic process which synchronously and uniformly involves the entire peripheral lymphoid system.

The lack of any detectable effect of RTI monotherapy on viral load in lymph nodes of HIV-infected patients in early stage disease indicates the need for more potent antiviral regimens in this setting. In this regard, similar studies utilizing combination therapy including nucleoside analogues and protease inhibitors will be instructive. Analysis of lymph node biopsy samples from patients with moderately advanced HIV disease before and 8 weeks after adding a second RTI to an ongoing regimen of RTI monotherapy revealed decreases in viral replication in lymph node mononuclear cells which were paralleled by decreases in plasma viremia. Despite these significant decreases in measures of viral replication, the frequency of HIV-infected cells within lymph nodes remained essentially unchanged. From the perspective of pathogenesis, these data support the concept that most viral replication at any given time arises from a relatively small fraction of newly infected cells. As potent combinations of antiretroviral agents are tested, it will be essential to monitor their effects on critical parameters involved in HIV pathogenesis such as viral trapping within germinal centers, the frequency of HIV-infected cells (i.e., viral burden) within lymphoid tissue, and viral replication within cells in lymphoid tissue.

Acknowledgement. The authors acknowledge the contributions of Dr. Cecil Fox, Dr. Jan Orenstein, and Mary Rust. Studies discussed in this review were part of the Division of AIDS Treatment Research Initiative (DATRI). The contributions of the DATRI 003 study team are gratefully acknowledged (see [9, 44]).

References

1. Fauci A, Schnittman S, Poli G, Koenig S, Pantaleo G (1991) Immunopathogenic mechanisms in human immunodeficiency virus (HIV) infection. Ann Intern Med 114:678
2. Bagnarelli P, Menzo S, Valenza A, et al (1992) Molecular profile of human immunodeficiency virus type 1 infection in symptomless patients and in patients with AIDS. J Virol 66:7328
3. Piatak M, Saag M, Yang L, et al (1993) High levels of HIV-1 in plasma during all stages of infection determined by competitive PCR. Science 259:1749
4. Pantaleo G, Graziosi C, Butini L, et al (1991) Lymphoid organs function as major reservoirs for human immunodeficiency virus. Proc Natl Acad Sci USA 88:9838
5. Pantaleo G, Graziosi C, Demarest JF, et al (1993) HIV infection is active and progressive in lymphoid tissue during the clinically latent stage of disease. Nature 362:355
6. Embretson J, Zupancic M, Ribas J, et al (1993) Massive covert infection of helper T lymphocytes and macrophages by HIV during the incubation period of AIDS. Nature 362:359
7. Wei X, Ghosh SK, Taylor ME, et al (1995) Viral dynamics in human immunodeficiency virus type 1 infection. Nature 373:117
8. Ho DD, Neumann AU, Perelson AS, Chen W, Leonard JM, Markowitz M (1995) Rapid turnover of plasma virions and CD4 lymphocytes in HIV-1 infection. Nature 373:123
9. Cohen OJ, Pantaleo G, Holodniy M, et al (1995) Decreased HIV-1 plasma viremia during antiretroviral therapy reflects downregulation of viral replication in lymphoid tissue. Proc Natl Acad Sci USA 1995, 92:6017
10. Mondino A, Khoruts A, Jenkins M (1996) The anatomy of T-cell activation and tolerance. Proc Natl Acad Sci USA 93:2245
11. Pantaleo G, Graziosi C, Demarest JF, Cohen O, Vaccarezza M, Gantt K, et al (1994) Role of lymphoid organs in the pathogenesis of human immunodeficiency virus (HIV) infection. Immunol Rev 140:105
12. Koup RA, Safrit JT, Cao Y, et al (1994) Temporal association of cellular immune responses with the initial control of viremia in primary human immunodeficiency virus type 1 syndrome. J Virol 68:4650
13. Borrow P, Lewicki H, Hahn BH, Shaw GM, Oldstone MB (1994) Virus-specific CD8[+] cytotoxic T-lymphocyte activity associated with control of viremia in primary human immunodeficiency virus type 1 infection. J Virol 68:6103
14. Joling P, Bakker L, Van Strijp J, et al (1993) Binding of human immunodeficiency virus type-1 to follicular dendritic cells in vitro is complement dependent. J Immunol 150:1065

15. Spiegel H, Herbst H, Niedobitek G, Foss H, Stein H (1992) Follicular dendritic cells are a major reservoir for human immunodeficiency virus type 1 in lymphoid tissues facilitating infection of CD4+ T-helper cells. Am J Pathol 140:15

16. Rácz P, Tenner-Rácz K, Kahl C, et al (1986) Spectrum of morphologic changes of lymph nodes from patients with AIDS or AIDS-related complexes. Prog Allergy 37:81

17. Turner R, Levine A, Gill P, Parker J, Meyer P (1987) Progressive histopathologic abnormalities in the persistent generalized lymphadenopathy syndrome. Am J Surg Pathol 11:625

18. Sei S, Akiyoshi H, Bernard J, et al (1996) Dynamics of virus versus host interaction in children with human immunodeficiency virus type 1 infection. J Infect Dis 173:1485

19. Heath SL, Tew JG, Tew JG, Szakal AK, Burton GF (1995) Follicular dendritic cells and human immunodeficiency virus infectivity. Nature 377:740

20. Bukrinsky M, Stanwick T, Dempsey M, Stevenson M (1991) Quiescent T lymphocytes as an inducible virus reservoir in HIV-1 infection. Science 254:423

21. Ascher M, Sheppard H (1988) AIDS as immune system activation: a model for pathogenesis. Clin Exp Immunol 73:165

22. Bass H, Nishanian P, Hardy W, et al (1992) Immune changes in HIV infection: significant correlations and differences in serum markers and lymphoid phenotypic antigens. Clin Immunol Immunopathol 64:63

23. Sheppard HW, Ascher MS, McRae B, Anderson RE, Lang W, Allain JP (1991) The initial immune response to HIV and immune system activation determine the outcome of HIV disease. J Acquir Immune Defic Syndr 4:704

24. Fauci A (1988) The human immunodeficiency virus: infectivity and mechanisms of pathogenesis. Science 239:617

25. Fauci A (1993) Multifactorial nature of human immunodeficiency virus diseases: implications for therapy. Science 262:1011

26. Rosenberg Z, Fauci A (1989) Induction of expression of HIV in latently or chronically infected cells. AIDS Res Hum Retroviruses 5:1

27. Poli G, Fauci AS (1993) Cytokine modulation of HIV expression. Semin Immunol 5:165

28. Graziosi C, Pantaleo G, Gantt KR, et al (1994) Lack of evidence for the dichotomy of TH1 and TH2 predominance in HIV-infected individuals. Science 265:248

29. Zack JA, Arrigo SJ, Weitsman SR, Go AS, Haislip A, Chen IS (1990) HIV-1 entry into quiescent primary lymphocytes: molecular analysis reveals a labile, latent viral structure. Cell 61:213

30. Westermann J, Persin S, Matyas J, Meide P van der, Pabst R (1994) Migration of so-called naive and memory T lymphocytes from blood to lymph in the rat. The influence of IFN-gamma on the circulation pattern. J Immunol 152:1744

31. Sprenger R, Toellner K, Schmetz C, et al (1995) Follicular dendritic cells productively infected with immunodeficiency viruses transmit infection to T cells. Med Microbiol Immunol 184:129

32. Schmitz J, Lunzen J van, Tenner-Racz K, et al (1994) Follicular dendritic cells retain HIV-1 particles on their plasma membrane, but are not productively infected in asymptomatic patients with follicular hyperplasia. J Immunol 153:1352

33. Hivroz C, Mazerolles F, Soula M, et al (1993) Human immunodeficiency virus gp120 and derived peptides activate protein tyrosine kinase p56lck in human CD4 T lymphocytes. Eur J Immunol 23:600

34. Goldman F, Jensen W, Johnson G, Heasley L, Cambier J (1994) gp120 ligation of CD4 induces p56lck activation and TCR desensitization independent of TCR tyrosine phosphorylation. J Immunol 153:2905

35. Banda N, Bernier J, Kurahara D, et al (1992) Cross-linking CD4 by human immunodeficiency virus gp120 primes T cells for activation-induced apoptosis. J Exp Med 176:1099

36. Li C, Friedman D, Wang C, Metelev V, Pardee A (1995) Induction of apoptosis in uninfected lymphocytes by HIV-1 tat protein. Science 268:429

37. Westendorp M, Frank R, Ochsenbauer C, et al (1995) Sensitization of T cells to CD95-mediated apoptosis by HIV-1 tat and gp120. Nature 375:497

38. Howcroft T, Strebel K, Martin M, Singer D (1993) Repression of MHC class I gene promoter activity by two-exon tat of HIV. Science 260:1320

39. Dawson V, Dawson T, Uhl G, Snyder S (1993) Human immunodeficiency virus type 1 coat protein neurotoxicity mediated by nitric oxide in primary cortical cultures. Proc Natl Acad Sci USA 90:3256

40. Pietraforte D, Tritarelli E, Testa U, Minetti M (1994) gp120 HIV envelope glycoprotein increases the production of nitric oxide in human monocyte-derived macrophages. J Leukoc Biol 55:175

41. Bukrinsky M, Nottet H, Schmidtmayerova H, et al (1995) Regulation of nitric oxide synthase activity in human immunodeficiency virus type 1 (HIV-1)-infected monocytes: implications for HIV-associated neurological disease. J Exp Med 181:735

42. Weeks B, Klotman M, Holloway E, Stetler-Stevenson W, Kleinman H, Klotman P (1993) HIV-1 infection stimulates T cell invasiveness and synthesis of the 92-kDa type IV collagenase. AIDS Res Hum Retroviruses 9:513

43. Lafrenie R, Wahl L, Epstein J, Hewlett I, Yamada K, Dhawan S (1996) HIV-1 tat modulates the function of monocytes and alters their interactions with microvessel endothelial cells. J Immunol 156:1638

44. Cohen O, Pantaleo G, Holodniy M, et al (1996) Antiretroviral monotherapy in early human immunodeficiency virus disease has no detectable effect on viral load in peripheral blood and lymph nodes. J Infect Dis 173:849

45. Biberfeld P, Chayt K, Marselle L, Biberfeld G, Gallo R, Harper M (1986) HTLV-III expression in infected lymph nodes and relevance to pathogenesis of lymphadenopathy. Am J Pathol 125:436

46. Fox C, Tenner-Rácz K, Rácz P, Firpo A, Pizzo P, Fauci A (1991) Lymphoid germinal centers are reservoirs of human immunodeficiency virus type 1 RNA. J Infect Dis 164:1051

47. Burke AP, Anderson D, Mannan P, et al (1994) Systemic lymphadenopathic histology in human immunodeficiency virus-1-seropositive drug addicts without apparent acquired immunodeficiency syndrome. Hum Pathol 25:248

48. Fischl M, Richman D, Grieco M, et al (1987) The efficacy of azidothymidine (AZT) in the treatment of patients with AIDS and AIDS-related complex. A double-blind, placebo-controlled trial. N Engl J Med 317:185

49. Fischl M, Richman D, Hansen N, et al (1990) The safety and efficacy of zidovudine (AZT) in the treatment of subjects with mildly symptomatic human immunodeficiency virus type 1 (HIV) infection. A double-blind, placebo-controlled trial. Ann Intern Med 112:727

50. Volberding P, Lagakos S, Koch M, et al (1990) Zidovudine in asymptomatic human immunodeficiency virus infection. A controlled trial in persons with fewer than 500 CD4$^-$ positive cells per cubic millimeter. N Engl J Med 322:941

51. Volberding P, Lagakos S, Grimes J, et al (1994) The duration of zidovudine benefit in persons with asymptomatic HIV infection. J Am Med Assoc 272:437

52. Vella S, Giuliano M, Dally L, et al (1994) Long-term follow-up of zidovudine therapy in asymptomatic HIV infection: results of a multicenter cohort study. J Acquir Immune Defic Syndr 7:31

53. Cooper D, Gatell J, Kroon S, et al (1993) Zidovudine in persons with asymptomatic HIV infection and CD4$^+$ cell counts greater than 400 per cubic millimeter. N Engl J Med 329:297

54. Concorde Coordinating Committee (1994) Concorde: MRC/ANRS randomised double-blind controlled trial of immediate and deferred zidovudine in symptom-free HIV infection. Lancet 343:871

55. Volberding P, Lagakos S, Grimes J, et al (1995) A comparison of immediate with deferred zidovudine therapy for asymptomatic HIV- infected adults with CD4 cell counts of 500 or more per cubic millimeter. N Engl J Med 333:401

56. Choi S, Lagakos S, Schooley R, Volberding P (1993) CD4$^+$ lymphocytes are an incomplete surrogate marker for clinical progression in persons with asymptomatic HIV infection taking zidovudine. Ann Intern Med 118:674

57. Armstrong J, Horne R (1984) Follicular dendritic cells and virus-like particles in AIDS-related lymphadenopathy. Lancet II:370

58. Baroni C, Pezzella F, Mirolo M, Ruco L, Rossi G (1986) Immunohistochemical demonstration of p24 HTLV-III major core protein in different cell types within lymph nodes from patients with lymphadenopathy syndrome (LAS). Histopathology 10:5

59. Lafeuillade A, Poggi C, Profizi N, Tamalet C, Costes O (1996) Human immunodeficiency virus type 1 kinetics in lymph nodes compared with plasma. J Infect Dis 174:404

60. Mellors J Jr, CR, Gupta P, White R, Todd J, Kingsley L (1996) Prognosis in HIV-1 infection predicted by the quantity of virus in plasma. Science 272:1167

61. O'Brien W, Hartigan P, Martin D, et al (1996) Changes in plasma HIV-1 RNA and CD4$^+$ lymphocyte counts and the risk of progression to AIDS. N Engl J Med 334:426

62. Sei S, Kleiner D, Kopp J, et al (1994) Quantitative analysis of viral burden in tissues from adults and children with symptomatic human immunodeficiency virus type 1 infection assessed by polymerase chain reaction. J Infect Dis 170:325

63. Perrin L, Yerly S, Lazzarin A, et al (1996) Reduced viremia and increased CD4/CD8 ratio in patients with primary HIV infection treated with AZT-ddI. Eleventh International Conference on AIDS, Vancouver, 1996. We.B. 532
64. Markowitz M, Cao Y, Hurley A, et al (1996) Triple therapy with AZT, 3TC, and ritonavir in 12 subjects newly infected with HIV-1. Eleventh International Conference on AIDS, Vancouver, 1996. Th.B. 933
65. Saimot AG, Simon F, Landman R, et al (1996) A triple nucleoside analogue combination in four patients with primary HIV-1 infections: towards complete virological remissions? Eleventh International Conference on AIDS, Vancouver, 1996. Mo.B. 1332
66. Kinloch-De Loes S, Hirschel BJ, Hoen B, et al (1995) A controlled trial of zidovudine in primary human immunodeficiency virus infection. N Engl J Med 333:408
67. Perelson AS, Essungen P, Markowitz M, Ho DD (1996) How long should treatment be given if we had an antiretroviral regimen that completely blocks HIV replication? Eleventh International Conference on AIDS, Vancouver, 1996. Th.B. 930

Mechanisms of resistance to HIV infection

William A. Paxton, Richard A. Koup

Aaron Diamond AIDS Research Center and the Rockefeller University, 455 First Avenue, 7th Floor, New York, NY 10016, USA

Introduction

The global expansion of the HIV-1 pandemic represents one of the world's most pressing public health problems. HIV-1 has spread from the sites of the original epidemic in Africa, North America and Europe to involve all corners of the globe. This includes the rapid and devastating spread of HIV-1 into human populations in India, Southeast Asia, and South America. The vast majority of new HIV-1 infections worldwide occur through sexual contact. The second most common route of transmission is from mother to infant during pregnancy and delivery, or after birth as a result of breast feeding. In comparison to these routes of transmission, the worldwide incidence of new HIV-1 infections from direct intravenous injection of contaminated blood, either via medical administration of contaminated blood products or from sharing of needles during the recreational use of intravenously injected drugs, is almost negligible.

The risk of an individual becoming infected with HIV-1 generally varies with the route, magnitude, and frequency of exposure. The highest rates of transmission after a single exposure are reported in recipients of contaminated blood products [11, 105]. It is rare that the transfusion of a single unit of contaminated packed red blood cells to a seronegative donor has not resulted in transmission of HIV-1. When transfusion of contaminated blood products does not result in transmission, it can usually be ascribed to a very low viral load within the particular preparation [11]. It is also obvious that inoculation of contaminated blood does not usually result in infection if the inoculum is very low, as occurs with most accidental needle stick injuries [71].

There is also an inoculum effect associated with transmission risk in maternal-fetal transmission of HIV-1. Several studies have demonstrated a correlation between the maternal virus load and risk of infection in the infant [7, 36, 40]. In addition, the administration of the antiretroviral agent zidovudine to the mother around the time of delivery, and to the newborn, resulted in a significant decrease in the rate of transmission [28]. The benefit, however, could not be entirely ascribed to a lowering

---

Correspondence to: W.A. Paxton

of the viral load in the mothers; some benefit may have come from the treatment of the infant [94]. There is other indirect evidence for the role of the virus inoculum in maternal-fetal transmission. During vaginal delivery of twins the first twin is more likely than the second twin to become infected with HIV-1, leading to speculation that the first twin to traverse the birth canal encounters the greatest amount of virus and also "cleanses" the canal for the second twin [42]. Infants delivered vaginally are more likely to become infected than are those delivered by cesarean section, possibly reflecting the lower exposure to maternal blood associated with the latter procedure [42, 100]. Transmission rates are also higher among infants where there was prolonged rupture of maternal membranes prior to delivery, suggesting they spent a prolonged time exposed to maternal virus [57].

Virus inoculum, however, is not the entire story in maternal-fetal transmission. Several studies have now demonstrated that there is not a maternal viral threshold above which transmission is likely to occur, making maternal viral load a poor predictor of transmission [10, 55, 94]. There is also evidence that maternal-fetal transmission does not fit a simple stochastic model; selection of certain genotypes and phenotypes of HIV-1 occurs during the transmission process [85, 107].

The overwhelming majority of new HIV-1 infections worldwide occur as a result of transmission during sexual intercourse. The factors affecting this mode of transmission, however, are not well studied. Measurements of virus load within sexual fluids, including vaginal secretions, pre-ejaculate and ejaculate, have been difficult to perform and of variable accuracy [4, 56, 65, 84]. Several epidemiologic studies, however, have shed light on the transmission process. Among homosexual men, the practice associated with the greatest risk of acquiring HIV-1 infection is receptive anal intercourse with an HIV-1-infected partner [51]. This risk is increased if trauma may have been induced by the prior insertion of other objects [18]. There also appears to be an association between the stage of the disease of the positive partner and the risk of transmission; the more immune compromised the donor, and by inference the higher the virus load, the more likely HIV-1 is to be transmitted [31]. These data suggest, though do not prove, that a high virus load within the seminal fluid, and trauma-induced damage to the rectal mucosa during the process of receptive anal intercourse, allow for the efficient transfer of HIV-1 between partners.

Heterosexual, not homosexual, contact is the dominant route of transmission worldwide. The risk of HIV-1 infection through a single heterosexual exposure has been estimated to be low [76, 83]. However, multiple factors may affect the overall risk of transmission including the number of exposures, the presence or absence of a foreskin on the male, the presence or absence of genital ulcer disease, and the presence or absence of other sexually transmitted diseases, among others [14, 38, 74, 81, 82, 93]. Again, the major determinants of infection risk appear to be the magnitude of the inoculum, both in terms of virus load and frequency of exposure, and the integrity of the mucosal barrier.

As in maternal-fetal transmission, studies of sexual transmission indicate that HIV-1 is not transmitted in accordance with a purely stochastic model. Extensive virologic analysis of sexually transmitted viruses, including studies on the virus donor, have indicated that selection of non-syncytium-inducing (NSI) viruses occurs during transmission, and that, within transmitted viruses, there is strong pressure to conserve amino acid sequences within the envelope glycoprotein as compared to the gag proteins [109–111]. One could speculate that virus load within the donor's sexual fluids and the integrity of the mucosal barrier within the recipient are the primary determinants of whether or not an adequate inoculum is delivered. The selection process helps determine what that inoculum must contain for transmission to occur; a large inoculum lacking the correct viral phenotype or genotype will not result in transmission, while a small inoculum containing the correct virus profile may be adequate for transmission.

Multiply exposed uninfected individuals

Despite the speed with which HIV-1 is spreading worldwide, there is increasing recognition that not all individuals who are extensively exposed to HIV-1 necessarily become infected. Indeed, multiple cohorts have been established and are being followed to determine the reasons behind the lack of seroconversion in certain high-risk individuals. These subjects fall into all exposure categories. Several patients with severe hemophilia have been identified who received large amounts of non-heat-treated factor VIII preparations during the early 1980s, yet failed to become infected [59, 67]. The lack of infection cannot be traced to non-receipt of certain lots of factor VIII. By all criteria these individuals should have become infected, but did not.

Less convincing as epidemiologic outlyers, though still of interest, are the 80% of infants born to HIV-1-infected mothers who fail to acquire that infection [72]. Do some or all of these infants resist infection despite exposure to maternal blood, or are most of them simply exposed to a sub-optimal inoculum? Further study of these infants would be prudent, especially since it has recently been suggested that HIV-1 infection can resolve in some infants, indicating an active process of resistance to infection [5, 9, 86]. It will also be important in the future to sort out true episodes of viral clearance from possible laboratory contaminations [53, 73].

Sexually active homosexual men account for many of the high-risk seronegative patients studied to date. The exposure histories are often variable within and between different populations that have all been defined as highly exposed but uninfected, and this has occasionally led to discrepant results when different cohorts were studied. For instance, when exposed-uninfected subjects were identified through the Multicenter AIDS Cohort Study (MACS), many of these subjects were found to have "silent" or antibody-negative infections [45]. Follow-up studies had difficulty confirming these initial observations [44], and when other investigators looked for the same phenomenon in their own cohorts, variable results were obtained [8, 30, 54, 78]. It is, therefore, important to remember that no two individuals have the exact same exposure history, nor do two cohorts have the same definition of high-risk exposure, and these facts may affect the statistical power and conclusions of different studies. It should also be noted that several cohorts have been established in the USA to study both homosexual and heterosexual couples that are sexually active yet remain discordant for HIV infection. Since the HIV-infected partner is known for each exposed-uninfected subject in these cohorts, it allows for the comprehensive evaluation of virologic and host factors in both the infected and uninfected partner, where other cohorts can only study the uninfected partner.

From an epidemiologic standpoint, the most impressive subjects are from the cohorts of female commercial sex workers in Africa [101]. In one cohort of prostitutes in Nairobi, Kenya, 50% of women entering the trade seroconverted in the 1st year. However, the rate of seroconversion did not remain constant in the cohort. Approximately 5% of the prostitutes remained seronegative no matter how long they had been

Table 1. Proposed mechanisms for resistance to HIV-1 infection

I Stochastic
    Chance alone
II Acquisition of immunity
    Cellular
        Class I-restricted CTL (local or systemic)
        Class II-restricted Th (local or systemic)
        CD8 cell antiviral factors[a]
    Humoral
        Local mucosal B cell immunity
        Systemic low frequency B cell immunity
        Antibody to MHC
III Innate resistance
    Genetic
        CC CKR-5 polymorphism
        Factors linked to the MHC locus
        β-chemokine production

CTL, Cytotoxic T lymphocytes; Th, T helper (cell); MHC, major histocompatibility complex
[a]Some CD8 cell antiviral activity is associated with the action of the β-chemokines, and both may be operative as acquired or innate responses

practicing prostitution. These women did not differ from the rest of the cohort in terms of sexual practices, number of contacts, or condom use. Epidemiologically they can be defined as resisting HIV-1 infection. How this occurs, however, is unclear.

Multiple potential mechanisms have been proposed to account for lack of HIV-1 transmission in exposed-uninfected individuals. A non-comprehensive list is provided in Table 1. In the following sections, we will discuss the evidence in support of several of these mechanisms.

Mechanisms of resistance: cell-mediated immunity

A vaccine for HIV-1 is a much needed necessity. Despite recent successes with combination anti-retroviral chemotherapy, the high costs of these agents makes it unlikely that they will be used in the developing countries of the world, where HIV-1 infection is most prolific. A vaccination strategy is clearly needed which will provide long-term immunity against the multiple and variant clades of both HIV-1 and -2. How realistic a goal this is remains to be determined. Before such a vaccine can be developed, a better understanding of the correlates of immunity may be required. Studying those individuals who have acquired natural immunity to HIV-1, i.e., those individuals who have been multiply exposed to replicating virus but who have not become infected, is one way of dissecting these correlates. The identification of protective immune responses in such individuals would indicate what is required from a vaccine and what immune responses should be provoked.

Since all individuals recruited into such exposed-uninfected studies are HIV-1 antibody negative, it can be assumed that it is not a B cell response against HIV-1 antigen that is protecting these individuals from infection unless, of course, it is a localized or low-frequency response [46]. Indeed, while it cannot be stated with certainty that HIV-1-specific B cells and mucosal IgA responses to HIV-1 are absent in exposed-uninfected individuals, their presence has not been proven. The absence of a detectable antibody response following viral exposure does not necessarily indicate an absence of protective immunity. Indeed, both major histocompatability complex (MHC) class I and class II responses have been identified in exposed but uninfected individuals. Stimulation of T cell immunity, in the absence of B cell immunity, could occur through exposure to low levels of HIV-1.

Cellular immune responses to viruses are varied and complex. Various viral infections are controlled by $CD8^+$ cytotoxic T lymphocytes (CTL) which recognize peptide antigen associated with the MHC class 1 molecule [12, 68, 92, 108]. T helper (Th) responses are mediated by $CD4^+$ lymphocytes which recognize antigen in the context of the MHC class II molecule [91]. The $CD4^+$ Th response is split between that of Th1 and Th2, both of which can be categorized by cytokine secretory profiles [16, 34, 75, 89]. Th1 lymphocytes predominantly secrete interleukin (IL)-2 and interferon-γ (IFN-γ) which can enhance the cell-mediated effector arm of the immune response (such as the CTL), while Th2 cells predominantly secrete IL-4, IL-5, IL-6 and IL-10, which enhance the B cell effector arm [16, 34, 75, 89]. Both Th1 and Th2 responses can down-regulate each other via cytokine-mediated mechanisms [89]. These Th cytokine secretory profiles are not absolute, but they do provide a means for analyzing the immune response.

It has been suggested that a predominant Th1 response could be operative in exposed-uninfected individuals, with a strong Th1 response eliciting a protective CTL response, while simultaneously down-modulating HIV-1-specific antibody production.

Reports of Th responses in exposed-uninfected individuals have been published [20–22, 25, 49]. One study demonstrated that peripheral blood mononuclear cells (PBMC) from exposed-uninfected individuals secreted IL-2 when stimulated in vitro with recombinant HIV-1 envelope (env) antigen and peptides [21, 22]. PBMC from six out of six gay men at risk of HIV-1 infection showed higher levels of IL-2 secretion upon env stimulation than PBMC from control individuals. These findings were followed by a report describing HIV-1 antigen-reactive Th responses in a group of health care workers who had been exposed to HIV-1 through needle stick injuries [25]. A similar observation was reported for a group of infants born to HIV-1-infected mothers, suggesting that an env-specific Th response may protect against vertical transmission of HIV-1 [23]. In all of the studies described above, it was a Th1 response which was preferentially activated in the exposed individuals; IL-2 was produced in vitro. This led to the speculation that exposed individuals who had developed an early and strong Th1-type response to HIV-1 were at least partially protected. However, to establish the protective effect of the Th1 response, they would have to be shown to be absent from individuals who became infected as a result of their exposure. A T cell proliferative response to HIV-1 antigen indicates that a memory response has been established and, therefore, one should be able to detect the end result of this activity, such as antibody production or CTL induction. The inability to detect such responses in the blood of exposed individuals may reflect the localized nature of the immune response. A Th response may be induced and be detectable systemically, but the B cell or CTL response may be localized to the inductive site; the mucosal surface or the regional draining lymphoid tissue. The ability of a Th1 response to protect against HIV-1 is supported by the finding that progressive loss of $CD4^+$ lymphocytes during HIV-1 infection often occurs in association with a switch from a Th1 response to that of Th2, suggesting that a Th1 response may be involved in controlling HIV-1 replication [20].

The presence of a Th response is not indicative of exposure to live virus but may only reflect exposure to viral antigen in the form of defective viral particles.

The identification of a CD8$^+$ CTL response to HIV-1 would indicate that the individual had experienced active virus infection; viral antigen would have had to have been processed and presented via the MHC class 1 pathway. The identification of CTL activity in an uninfected individual would suggest that viral infection had been cleared, either spontaneously or as a result of the induced immune response. Several reports have now described such CTL activity in exposed-uninfected individuals [35, 58, 80, 87, 88]. A study by Langlade-Demoyen et al. [58] showed nef-specific CTL activity in a group of seronegative heterosexual partners of HIV-1-infected individuals. In another study of seronegative health care workers who were exposed to HIV-1 through a single occupational accident, env-specific CTL responses were demonstrated [80]. A report by Detels et al. [35] on HIV-1 highly exposed gay men also suggests that resistance to infection may be associated with a CD8$^+$ lymphocyte response. A comprehensive study by Rowland-Jones et al. [88] has described CTL responses in a cohort of seronegative commercial sex workers from the Gambia who were heavily exposed to HIV. Using peptides to restimulate low-level responses in vitro, they demonstrated HIV-1 pol- and nef-specific, HLA-B35 class I-restricted responses in three of six exposed-seronegative women in comparison to no responses in the non-exposed, HLA-B35-matched control women [88]. The fact that peptide restimulations were required to detect the CTL responses suggests there was a limited precursor frequency of these memory cells. It is not known whether the presence of this induced CTL response simply reflects that there had been restricted viral infection at the site of exposure, presumably at the vaginal mucosa, or whether it was actually responsible for blocking viral dissemination. Another study by Rowland-Jones et al. [87] has identified transient gag-specific CTL activity in a child born to a HIV-1-infected mother. This child has remained negative for HIV-1 infection, suggesting that exposure to replicating virus may have induced a protective CTL response. Others have reported similar results in exposed-uninfected infants [1, 17, 32].

Further evidence for the role of cellular immunity in protection against HIV-1 infection comes from studies demonstrating a correlation between MHC profile and risk of seroconversion [47, 48, 50, 52, 97]. While the mechanism underlying these observations remain obscure, it is possible that expression of certain MHC molecules may affect the ability of some individuals to mount an immune response against HIV-1. It has also been noted within commercial sex workers in Nairobi, Kenya, that those expressing rare MHC alleles are the ones most likely to remain uninfected, suggesting that alloimmunity may provide protection. This concept is supported by studies demonstrating that class I and class II molecules are present on the surface of HIV-1 virions, and that macaques can be protected against human cell-grown simian immunodeficiency virus (SIV) when the animals had been previously vaccinated with fixed uninfected human cells [3, 15, 99].

Cell-mediated immune responses have also been identified in primate models of HIV-1 infection. Both rhesus macaques and chimpanzees have been shown to be protected against low-dose viral challenges with SIV and HIV, respectively, through the induction of mucosal immune responses [24, 90]. In one report, rhesus macaques were inoculated rectally with 100 infectious doses of SIV$_{mac251}$ and seroconverted, while the animals given a lower dose of 10 infectious doses did not seroconvert over a 2-year period. The monkeys who received the low dose of virus and who did not seroconvert remained seronegative when they were subsequently challenged with a higher viral inoculum [90]. These animals, when analyzed further, showed a greater in vitro proliferative response to SIV and a higher degree of CD8$^+$ cell-mediated SIV

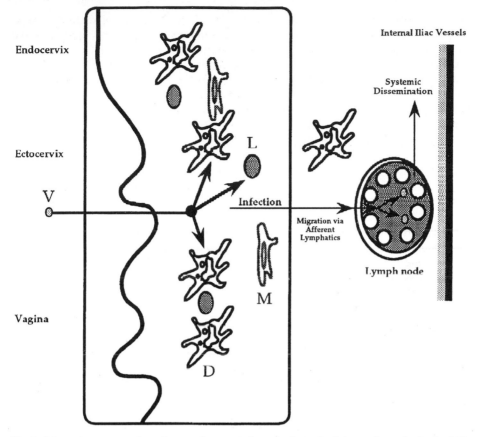

Fig. 1. Schematic representation of mucosal transmission of primate lentiviruses. Langerhan's dendritic cells (*D*), macrophages (*M*), lymphocytes (*L*), and virus (*V*) are shown in association with the epithelial layer, a regional draining lymph node, and the systemic circulation. Adapted from Spira et al. [96]

suppressor activity than the non-infected control animals [90]. The observed suppressor activity may or may not have been a reflection on class I-restricted CTL activity, and may or may not have been stimulated by the previous low-dose inoculation; both these points still need to be addressed. Another study with macaques demonstrated that low-dose mucosal inoculation resulted in protection from subsequent higher-dose SIV challenges [24]. This protection was also associated with the presence of SIV-specific proliferative responses in the absence of specific antibody [24]. These results are consistent with what has been identified in some exposed-uninfected humans. Another study has shown that antiviral CTL are present in the vaginal mucosa of SIV-infected rhesus macaques [66]. Although these monkeys were infected it does demonstrate that SIV-specific CTL can be induced in the vaginal epithelium of macaques; the site where such cells would be expected to be induced in exposed-seronegative individuals who have experienced localized, transient infection with HIV-1.

A recent study of vaginal inoculation of SIV into macaques has determined that the first cells to be infected are in the lamina propria of the cervicovaginal mucosa, immediately subjacent to the epithelium [96]. These infected cells appear to be antigen-presenting cells such as Langerhan's dendritic cells, and not lymphocytes or monocytes. The infection rapidly spreads to the regional draining lymph nodes prior to systemic dissemination. It was also apparent from this study that not all monkeys in whom a mucosal infection with SIV was established would be expected to develop disseminated infection, lending credence to the hypothesis that some exposed-seronegative humans may have experienced a transient localized infection at the mucosal site of inoculation in the absence of systemic infection. Figure 1 provides a picture of the local mucosal architecture, and the cells infected by primate lentiviruses in traversing this layer.

Macaques immunized with a SIV env and p27 subunit vaccine delivered to the iliac lymph nodes were recently shown to be protected against rectal, but not vaginal, challenge with SIV [60]. This study indicates that protection may be dependent on the site of vaccination, and suggests that dissemination of infection from the mucosal site to the periphery can be immunologically controlled within the regional draining lymph nodes. In agreement with other studies, the protection in this set of experiments was shown to be associated with the induction of Th responses. However, most of these animals also developed a detectable serum IgA and IgG response. Despite this difference between these animal studies and exposed-uninfected humans, the similarities are remarkable and suggest that exposure to HIV-1 viral antigen at a mucosal site of infection could protect against subsequent exposure to live virus at the same site [60].

Mechanisms of resistance: CD8 suppressor activity

For many years it has been known that $CD8^+$ lymphocytes can suppress HIV-1 replication in vitro through the secretion of soluble factors [13, 63, 104]. This $CD8^+$ lymphocyte-mediated inhibition of viral replication is non-cytolytic and is not MHC restricted [69], in contrast to the antiviral activity mediated by class I-restricted HIV-1-specific CTL. It has been speculated that the ability of PBMC to secrete $CD8^+$ antiviral factor (CAF) contributes to maintaining the low viral burdens associated with the asymptomatic phase of infection [13, 61, 63]. There have been studies which have tried to link the secretion of CAF with protection from infection in groups of exposed but uninfected individuals [69]. One report describes the presence of an active CAF response in a group of heterosexual HIV-1-seronegative individuals who are repeatedly exposed to HIV-1 through sexual activity with known HIV-1-infected sexual partners [69]. Another report describes a high incidence of such a response in a group of uninfected infants born to HIV-1-infected mothers [62]. These studies, however, did not determine the identity of the suppressor factor or factors, nor did they determine if the factors were stimulated by the previous exposure to HIV-1.

In December 1995, Cocchi et al. [27] reported the identification of a group of molecules that are secreted by $CD8^+$ lymphocyte and have high anti-HIV-1 activity. These molecules belonged to a group of cytokines known as β-chemokines. The three β-chemokines identified were macrophage inflammatory protein-1α (MIP-1α), MIP-1β and 'regulated upon activation normal T cell expressed and secreted' (RANTES). All three molecules individually possessed anti-HIV-1 activity but in combination proved to be highly effective at inhibiting HIV-1 replication. Chemokines can be sub-divided into two families; α-chemokines which have a characteristic C-X-C motif close to the N terminus of the 8-kDa polypeptide, and the β-chemokines which possess a C-C motif at the same position [43]. The normal physiologic function of these proteins is varied but generally encompasses such functions as induction of lymphocyte and monocyte chemotaxis and the regulation of inflammatory responses [43]. Only recently have the β-chemokines RANTES, MIP-1α and MIP-1β been shown to possess specific anti-HIV-1 suppressor properties. Their anti-HIV-1 activity, however, appears to be limited to primary HIV-1 isolates; they are incapable of suppressing T cell line-adapted (TCLA) viruses [27, 79].

Mechanisms of resistance: CD4 cell infectability

It is widely accepted that PBMC from different donors vary in their susceptibility to infection with HIV-1 in vitro [26, 95, 103, 106]. Our own group recently identified relative resistance of CD4$^+$ lymphocytes to HIV-1 infection in a cohort of 25 highly exposed but uninfected individuals [79]. This resistance to infection was restricted to primary isolates of HIV-1, which probably accounts for the fact that this observation had previously gone unreported; most laboratories had used TCLA viruses for such studies. Given that β-chemokines have been shown to inhibit primary HIV-1 isolates but not TCLA viruses, we looked for and found a correlation between high secretion of RANTES, MIP-1α and MIP-1β from purified CD4$^+$ lymphocytes from two of our most resistant donors (EU2 and EU3) when compared to two susceptible control individuals. The demonstration that purified CD4$^+$ lymphocytes from these two individuals secreted approximately a log more of the β-chemokines was thought to explain the inability of their lymphocytes to be infected with primary isolates of HIV-1. An interesting point to note is that purified CD8$^+$ lymphocytes from both EU2 and EU3 also secrete tenfold more RANTES, MIP-1α and MIP-1β than purified CD8$^+$ lymphocytes from control individuals (Paxton et al. unpublished data). CD8$^+$ lymphocytes from other individuals in our cohort of sexually exposed individuals possessed greater levels of CAF activity than the lymphocytes from our control subjects, and this CD8$^+$ inhibition occurred in the absence of a detectable cytotoxic response [79]. All of these results indicate that the antiviral activity of the β-chemokines, whether secreted from CD4$^+$ or CD8$^+$ cells, can be operative in protection against sexual transmission of HIV-1.

This phenomenon of decreased susceptibility to HIV-1 infection in vitro has been reported in other cohorts of exposed-uninfected subjects [59, 77]. One study involved a group of 16 patients with severe hemophilia who had been exposed to large quantities of non-heat-treated HIV-1-contaminated factor VIII concentrate [59]. In this study it was reported that the most highly exposed hemophiliacs had PBMC that were more resistant to in vitro infection with a pool of 20 primary HIV-1 isolates than PBMC from either moderately exposed or control individuals. Closer analysis of the restriction to infection, either by utilizing phenotypically distinct viral isolates or purified fractions of PBMC, is needed to better define the phenomenon in this population. A separate study was performed by Ometto et al. [77] in which HIV-1-uninfected infants born to HIV-1-infected mothers were used as the exposed-uninfected subjects [77]. In this study, viral isolates from the mothers were found to exhibit restricted growth on enriched CD4$^+$ lymphocytes from the corresponding infants. This same study also demonstrated that the viral phenotype played a role in the restricted replication of infant cells [77]. Furthermore, not all CD4$^+$ lymphocytes within an individual will have the same susceptibility to HIV-1 infection. The different Th subtypes of CD4$^+$ lymphocytes have been shown to possess different susceptibilities to infection with HIV-1 in vitro; Th1 cells are more resistant to HIV-1 infection than cells with the Th2 or Th0 cytokine secretory profile [70, 102]. The mechanism underlying this observation is as yet undefined.

Can much of the decreased infectability of CD4+ lymphocytes from exposed-uninfected subjects be ascribed to the β-chemokines, and if so, what is their mechanism of action against HIV-1? The initial indication that β-chemokines may be involved came from the findings of Cocchi et al. [27] that β-chemokines were only active against primary strains and not TCLA strains of HIV-1 [27]. This fitted with our observation that CD4+ lymphocytes from some of our exposed-uninfected subjects were resistant to infection with only primary isolates of HIV-1, and they secreted approximately a log more of all three β-chemokines. While these data only provided coincidental evidence of a linkage, it was quite compelling. We determined that the block to viral replication in the CD4+ cells from our resistant subjects, and that mediated by the β-chemokines both occurred at entry [39]. Further, it was determined that the β-chemokines functioned by blocking viral fusion, again in a primary isolate-specific manner, and that CD4+ lymphocytes from EU2 and EU3 would not fuse with cells expressing primary isolate envelopes [39]. At around the same time, it was revealed that a co-receptor required for entry of TCLA strains of HIV-1 had been cloned and identified as a seven-transmembrane G-coupled protein known as fusin [41]. What was striking about this discovery was that fusin and the β-chemokine receptors are both members of the same receptor superfamily. The implication was obvious that the β-chemokines identified by Cocchi et al. [27], and those associated with our exposed-uninfected subjects [79], could well be functioning by blocking a co-receptor used by primary isolates of HIV-1. It seemed more than feasible that different proteins from the same superfamily could be utilized for entry by primary and TCLA viruses. This observation quickly led to the discovery that the CC CKR-5 chemokine receptor molecule could function as a co-receptor for macrophage-tropic, or primary NSI, HIV-1 isolates [39]. At the same time four other groups reported on the ability of CC CKR-5 to function as a co-receptor for HIV entry, and some of these groups also reported that CC CKR-3 and CC CKR-2b could function in a similar capacity, albeit for a more restricted group of viruses [2, 19, 33, 37, 39].

What then was mediating the lack of primary isolate entry and high level of β-chemokine production in CD4+ lymphocytes from some exposed-uninfected subjects? There are numerous possible explanations for these findings including binding of endogenously expressed β-chemokines to the CC CKR-5 receptor resulting in receptor blocking prior to surface expression, down-regulation of the receptor molecule via feedback control from the high level of endogenously produced β-chemokine, or the presence of a defective receptor molecule leading to both lack of viral entry and increased β-chemokine production through lack of feedback control.

To address these various possibilities, the CC CKR-5 molecule from our two most resistant subjects, EU2 and EU3, were cloned and expressed. There was no entry of macrophage-tropic viruses into CD4-expressing 293T cells that had been transiently transfected with the CC CKR-5 from either individual, while there was entry of macrophage-tropic viruses if control CC CKR-5 was used [64]. The DNA sequence of the gene from these individuals revealed a homozygous 32-nucleotide base pair (bp) defect [64]. This 32-bp deletion lies within the second extracellular loop disrupting the reading frame of the protein, resulting in a truncated receptor which is not detectable at the cell surface. Lymphocytes from these individuals do not respond by Ca^{2+} flux to exogenous MIP-1β but do respond to RANTES, suggesting that other β-chemokine receptors are functional [64]. One parent each from EU2 and EU3 were studied and found to be heterozygous for the deletion, suggesting this to be an established allele within the population and not a mutational hotspot. This is supported by the fact that the deletion has been identical in all the cases found so far. Random sampling of genomic DNA from a European population revealed that 20% were heterozygous for the deletion. From this it can be predicted that 1% of similar European populations may be homozygous for the defective CC CKR-5 receptor [64]. On sampling 46 individuals from a Venezuelan population, no deletions were detected [64]. This observed variation in the frequency of the CC CKR-5 deletion between different ethnic groups may have an influence on the transmission rates of HIV throughout the world.

A defective CC CKR-5 receptor can explain the findings in EU2 and EU3, but it may not explain what is happening in exposed-uninfected subjects whose CD4$^+$ lymphocytes are only moderately resistant to HIV-1 infection. It is possible that the CC CKR-5 gene is highly polymorphic and some polymorphisms may affect the efficiency with which CC CKR-5 can function as a the co-receptor for HIV-1 entry. We and others are presently scrutinizing the CC CKR-5 molecule from moderately resistant individuals.

Polymorphisms within the CC CKR-5 gene that correlate with infectivity of CD4$^+$ lymphocytes in vitro may be important in more than just HIV-1 transmission. These polymorphisms may also affect efficiency of HIV-1 replication in vivo, thereby affecting virus load and rates of disease progression. Individuals who are heterozygous for the deleted CC CKR-5 gene may express low levels of CC CKR-5 on their cells' surface. If the expression of this co-receptor is limiting for viral entry, then there may be decreased efficiency of HIV-1 infection in heterozygous individuals, leading to an effect on the transmission and pathogenesis of HIV-1. Unfortunately, it is currently not possible to determine surface expression levels of the CC CKR-5 molecule on CD4$^+$ lymphocytes due to the lack of specific antibodies. Mechanisms notwithstanding, it will be important to determine whether there is a higher frequency of heterozygous individuals within exposed-uninfected populations and long-term nonprogressing subjects than in comparable control populations.

Despite these recent discoveries, many questions remain unanswered. Do CD4$^+$ lymphocytes from individuals who are heterozygous for the deleted CC CKR-5 gene exhibit intermediate infectability by HIV-1 due to co-receptor blockage by higher levels of endogenously secreted β-chemokines, or through decreased co-receptor expression on the cell surface? Does exposure to HIV-1 antigen or other pathogens, as would be predictably encountered through high-risk sexual behavior, modulate β-chemokine secretion from CD4$^+$ or CD8$^+$ lymphocytes? What is responsible for the up-regulation of β-chemokine secretion levels in the CD4$^+$ lymphocytes isolated from EU2 and EU3 and how this is mediated? What are the immunologic consequences of lacking functional CC CKR-5?

What does the CC CKR-5 co-receptor have to do with HIV-1 sexual transmission? If an individual possesses either a defective or blocked co-receptor then it is unlikely that an initial infection with HIV-1 can occur. The tissue expression patterns of CC CKR-5 within the mucosa are currently unknown, but will have obvious implications for transmission. Macrophages, as well as CD4$^+$ lymphocytes, from both EU2 and EU3 are refractory for infection with primary isolates of HIV-1 [29]. This suggests that HIV-1 utilizes the CC CKR-5 molecule not only on CD4$^+$ lymphocytes but on other cell types present within the vaginal and rectal mucosa that may be infected early during sexual transmission. It is unclear why primary NSI viral isolates are preferentially transmitted sexually when compared to the more virulent SI viral forms [110]. It is possible, however, that expression of different co-receptors on cells present within the mucosa may partially explain this observation. CC CKR-5, and not fusin, may be preferentially expressed on Langerhan's cells of the mucosa, thereby affording NSI isolates a selective transmission advantage over SI isolates.

The CD4$^+$ lymphocyte clones generated from our exposed-uninfected individuals also appear to be less infectable with TCLA viruses than the clones from the controls [39]. This would suggest that a relative resistance to infection via the fusin receptor may also occur. Exposure to multiple pathogens and or foreign MHC molecules may alter the β-chemokine secretion profiles or β-chemokine receptor expression levels at the site of exposure, thereby influencing HIV-1 transmission. Whether exposed-uninfected individuals possess high expression of β-chemokines in vivo as well as in vitro remains to be determined.

Even though an individual may express dysfunctional CC CKR-5, viral entry into antigen-presenting cells or other cells may occur through CD4-independent pathways [6, 98]. Therefore, the establishment of a localized infection may still be possible in an individual lacking a functional co-receptor, though dissemination of primary NSI isolates to CD4$^+$ lymphocytes in the regional draining lymph nodes would not occur. The localized infection within the mucosa might then enable the infected individual to develop an active, and possibly localized, cellular immune response against HIV-1. In individuals with polymorphisms that limit the ability of CC CKR-5 to act efficiently as a HIV-1 co-receptor, limited susceptibility of CD4$^+$ lymphocytes to HIV-1 infection and the induction of specific local immunity may combine to provide protection against transmission.

Conclusions

It is evident that no one single phenomenon will explain the apparent resistance to HIV-1 infection that has been observed in some highly exposed individuals. While lack of infection in some of these individuals may be explained purely by chance, it is clear that others have specific mechanisms that are providing some degree of protection. In some, such as those who are homozygous for a defective HIV-1 co-receptor gene, the degree of protection will likely be quite profound. In others, such as those who have generated localized or systemic immune responses to HIV-1, the degree of protection from subsequent infection is currently unknown. The architecture of the mucosa and the presence, within this tissue layer, of cells expressing CD4 and HIV-1 co-receptors CC CKR-5 and fusin, the secretion of the natural ligands for these receptors that can block HIV-1 infection, and the generation of specific immune responses, may all combine to influence the efficiency of transmission.

Individuals who do not express functional CC CKR-5, due to homozygous inheritance of a defect in this gene, resist infection because primary NSI isolates are unable to enter and establish infection within the mucosa. Theoretically, however, infection could be established with viruses that utilize other chemokine receptors as co-receptors. In the latter case, it is possible that a class I-restricted immune response could be generated locally, and in either case, a class II-restricted response could occur. It is probable, however, that the defect in CC CKR-5 is providing the bulk of the protection against infection in these individuals.

Resistance to infection may also occur in individuals who express other polymorphisms of CC CKR-5 or express high levels of β-chemokines that partially block the availability of CC CKR-5. In these individuals, if an initial mucosal infection is established, the efficiency of spread may be suboptimal. This could lead to viral clearance in conjunction with the stimulation of specific local immunity. A larger mucosal inoculum, however, may be able to overcome this resistance.

Finally, even individuals who do not exhibit any evidence of innate resistance, either in the form of CC CKR-5 polymorphisms or β-chemokine expression levels, may still resist infection. Exposure to low inocula of HIV-1 may be insufficient to result in disseminated infection, but may be sufficient to stimulate local immunity. It is also possible that local immunity, generated in response to previous challenge with an SI virus, which is naturally inefficient at establishing disseminated infection, could result in local immunity that would then protect against subsequent challenge with NSI viruses.

Further work is necessary to determine whether or not these scenarios are correct. In the interim, the bulk of data indicate that mucosal architecture, specific immune responses, β-chemokine production, and the genetics of the host, both with respect to the immune response and the function of HIV-1 co-receptors, combine in providing protection against mucosal transmission of HIV-1. This information should not be overlooked when considering vaccine design. Both the kind of immunity and the location of the immunity that should be stimulated by a vaccine might be inferred from studies on exposed-uninfected individuals. In addition, it must be considered that vaccines which specifically or non-specifically stimulate the local production of β-chemokines might also provide protection. Highly exposed, uninfected individuals remain an important group of subjects for intense study.

Acknowledgements. The authors thank Dr. Nathanial Landau, Dr. Rong Liu, Scott Martin, Sunny Choe, Daniel Ceradini, and Stan Kang for their multiple contributions to this work. We also thank Jovino Guza and Wendy Chen for assistance with typing and graphics. This work was supported by grants and contracts from the National Institutes of Health, RO1 AI35522, RO1 AI38573, and NO1 AI45218. R.A.K. is an Elizabeth Glaser Scientist of the Pediatric AIDS Foundation.

References

1. Aldous MC, Watret KC, Mok JY, Bird AG, Froebel KS (1994) Cytotoxic T lymphocyte activity and CD8 subpopulations in children at risk of HIV infection. Clin Exp Immunol 97:61
2. Alkhatib G, Combadiere C, Broder CC, Feng Y, Kennedy PE, Murphy PM, Berger EA (1996) CC CKR5: a RANTES, MIP-1α, MIP-1β receptor as a fusion cofactor for macrophage-tropic HIV-1. Science 272:1955
3. Arthur LO, Bess JW Jr, Sowder RC II, Benveniste RE, Mann DL, Chermann JC, Henderson LE (1992) Cellular proteins bound to immunodeficiency viruses: implications for pathogenesis and vaccines. Science 258:1935
4. Bagasra O, Farzadegan H, Seshamma T, Oakes JW, Saah A, Pomerantz RJ (1994) Detection of HIV-1 proviral DNA in sperm from HIV-1-infected men. J Acquir Immune Defic Syndr 8:1669
5. Bakshi SS, Tetali S, Abrams EJ, Paul MO, Pahwa SG (1995) Repeatedly positive human immunodeficiency virus type 1 DNA polymerase chain reaction in human immunodeficiency virus-exposed seroreverting infants. Pediatr Infect Dis J 14:658
6. Bhat S, Spitalnik SL, Gonzalez-Scarano F, Silberberg DH (1991) Galactosyl ceramide or a derivative is an essential component of the neural receptor for human immunodeficiency virus type 1 envelope glycoprotein gp120. Proc Natl Acad Sci USA 88:7131

7. Borkowsky W, Krasinski K, Cao Y, Ho D, Pollack H, Moore T, Chen SH, Allen M, Tao PT (1994) Correlation of perinatal transmission of human immunodeficiency virus type 1 with maternal viremia and lymphocyte phenotypes. J Pediatr 125:345

8. Brettler DB, Somasundaran M, Forsberg AF, Krause E, Sullivan JL (1992) Silent HIV-1 infection: a rare occurence in a high risk heterosexual population. Blood 80:2396

9. Bryson YJ, Pang S, Wei LS, Dickover R, Diagne A, Chen ISY (1995) Clearance of HIV infection in a perinatally infected infant. N Engl J Med 332:833

10. Burchett SK, Kornegay J, Pitt J, Landesman S, Rosenblatt H, Hillyer G, Garcia P, Kalish L, Burns D, Davenney K, Lew J (1996) Assessment of maternal plasma HIV viral load as a correlate of vertical transmission. Abstracts of the 3rd Conference on Retroviruses and Opportunistic Infections. (Infectious Diseases Society of America for the Foundation for Retrovirology and Human Health) abstr. no. LB3

11. Busch MP, Operskalski EA, Mosley JW, Lee T-H, Henrard D, Herman S, Sachs DH, Harris M, Huang W, Stram DO (1996) Factors influencing human immunodeficiency virus type 1 transmission by blood transfusion. J Infect Dis 174:26

12. Byrne JA, Oldstone MBA (1984) Biology of cloned cytotoxic T lymphocytes specific for lymphocytic choriomeningitis virus: clearance of virus in vivo. J Virol 51:682

13. Cao Y, Qing L, Zhang LQ, Safrit JT, Ho DD (1994) Virological and immunological characterization of long-term survivors of HIV-1 infection. N Engl J Med 332:201

14. Celentano DD, Nelson KE, Suprasert S, Eiumtrakul S, Tulvatana S, Kuntolbutra S, Akarasewi P, Matanasarawoot A, Wright NH, Sirisopana N, Theetranont C (1996) Risk factors for HIV-1 seroconversion among young men in northern Thailand. JAMA 275:122

15. Chan W, Rodgers A, Hancock R, Taffs F, Kitchin P, Farrar G, Llew F (1992) Protection in SIV-vaccinated monkeys correlates with anti-HLA class I antibody responses. J Exp Med 176:1203

16. Cherwinski HM, Schumacher JH, Brown KD, Mosmann TR (1987) Two types of mouse helper T cell clone. J Exp Med 166:1229

17. Cheynier R, Langlade-Demoyen P, Marescot MR, Blanche S, Blondin G, Wain-Hobson S, Griscelli C, Vilmer E, Plata F (1992) Cytotoxic T lymphocyte responses in the peripheral blood of children born to human immunodeficiency virus-1-infected mothers. Eur J Immunol 22:2211

18. Chmiel J, Detels R, Kaslow RA, VanRaden M, Kingsley LA, Brookmeyer R, The Multicenter AIDS Cohort Study Group (1987) Factors associated with prevalent human immunodeficiency virus (HIV) infection in the Multicenter AIDS Cohort Study. Am J Epidemiol 126:568

19. Choe H, Farzan M, Sun Y, Sullivan N, Rollins B, Ponath PD, Wu L, Mackay CR, LaRosa G, Newman W, Gerard N, Gerard C, Sodroski J (1996) The β-chemokine receptors CCR3 and CCR5 facilitate infection by primary HIV-1 isolates. Cell 85:1135

20. Clerici M, Shearer GM (1993) A T_H1 T_H2 switch is a critical step in the etiology of HIV infection. Immunol Today 14:107

21. Clerici M, Berzosky JA, Shearer GM, Tacket CO (1991) Exposure to human immunodeficiency virus type 1-specific T helper cell responses before detection of infection by polymerase chain reaction and serum antibodies. J Infect Dis 164:178

22. Clerici M, Giorgi JV, Chou CC, Gudeman VK, Zack JA, Gupta P, Ho HN, Nishanian PG, Berzofsky JA, Shearer GM (1992) Cell-mediated immune response to human immunodeficiency virus (HIV) type-1 in seronegative homosexual men with recent sexual exposure to HIV-1. J Infect Dis 165:1012

23. Clerici M, Sison AV, Berzofsky JA, Rakusan TA, Brandt CD, Ellaurie M, Villa M, Colie C, Venzon DJ, Sewver JL, Shearer G (1993) Cellular immune factors associated with mother-to-infant transmission of HIV. J Acquir Immune Defic Syndr 7:1427

24. Clerici M, Clark EA, Polacino P, Axberg I, Kuller L, Casey NI, Morton WR, Shearer GM, Benveniste RE (1994) T cell proliferation to subinfectious SIV correlates with lack of infection after challenge of macaques. J Acquir Immune Defic Syndr 8:1391

25. Clerici M, Levin JM, Kessler HA, Harris A, Berzofsky JA, Landay AL, Shearer GM (1994) HIV-specific T helper activity in seronegative health care workers exposed to contaminated blood. JAMA 271:42

26. Cloyd MW, Moore BE (1990) Spectrum of biological properties of human immunodeficiency virus (HIV-1) isolates. Virology 174:103

27. Cocchi F, DeVico AL, Garzino-Demo A, Arya SK, Gallo RC, Lusso P (1995) Identification of RANTES, MIP-1 alpha, and MIP-1 beta as the major HIV-suppressive factors produced by CD8$^+$ T cells. Science 270:1811

28. Connor EM, Sperling RS, Gelber R, Kiselev P, Scott G, O'Sullivan MJ, VanDyke R, Bey M, Shearer W, Jacobson RL (1994) Reduction of maternal-infant transmission of human immunodeficiency virus type 1 with zidovudine treatment. Pediatric AIDS Clinical Trials Group Protocol 076 Study Group. N Engl J Med 331:1173

29. Connor RI, Paxton WA, Sheridan KE, Koup RA (1996) Macrophages and CD4[+] T-lymphocytes from two multiply exposed uninfected individuals resist infection with primary NSI isolates of human immunodeficiency virus type 1. J Virol (in press)

30. Coutlee F, Olivier C, Cassol S, Voyuer H, Kessous EA, Saint AP, He Y, Fauvel M (1994) Absence of prolonged immunosilent infection with human immunodeficiency virus in individuals with high-risk behavior. Am J Med 96:42

31. DeGruttola V, Seage GR, Mayer KH, Horsburgh CR (1989) Infectiousness of HIV between male homosexual partners. J Clin Epidemiol 42:849

32. De Maria A, Cirillo C, Moretta L (1994) Occurence of HIV-specific CTL activity in apparently uninfected children born to HIV-1 infected mothers. J Infect Dis 170:1296

33. Deng H, Liu R, Ellmeir W, Choe S, Unutmaz D, Burkhart M, DiMarzio P, Marmon S, Sutton RE, Hill CM, Davis CB, Peiper SC, Schall TJ, Littman DR, Landau NR (1996) Identification of a major co-receptor for primary isolates of HIV-1. Nature 381:661

34. DelPrete GF, De Carli M, Mastromauro C, Biagiotti R, Macchia D, Falagiani P, Ricci M, Romagnani S (1991) Purified protein derivative of *Mycobacterium tuberculosis* and excretory-secretory antigen(s) of *Toxocara canis* expand in vitro human T cells with stable and opposite (type 1 T helper or type 2 T helper) profile of cytokine production. J Clin Invest 88:346

35. Detels R, Liu Z, Hennessey K, Kan J, Visscher BR, Taylor JMG, Hoover DR, Rinaldo CR, Phair JP, Saah AJ, Giorgi JV (1994) Resistance to HIV-1 infection. J Acquir Immune Defic Syndr Hum Retrovirology 7:1263

36. Dickover RE, Garratty EM, Herman SA, Sim MS, Plaeger S, Boyer PJ, Keller M, Deveikis A, Stiehm ER, Bryson YJ (1996) Identification of levels of maternal HIV-1 RNA associated with risk of perinatal transmission. Effect of maternal zidovudine treatment on viral load. JAMA 275.599

37. Doranz BJ, Rucker J, Yanjie Y, Symth RJ, Samson M, Peiper SC, Parmentier M, Collman RG, Doms RW (1996) A dual-tropic primary HIV-1 isolate that uses fusin and the β-chemokine receptors CKR-5, CKR-3, and CKR-2b as fusion cofactors. Cell 85:1149

38. Downs AM, De Vicenzi I (1996) Probability of Heterosexual transmission of HIV: relationship to the number of unprotected sexual contacts. J Acquir Immune Defic Syndr Hum Retrovirolgoy 11:388

39. Dragic T, Litwin V, Allaway GP, Martin SR, Huang Y, Nagashima KA, Cayanan C, Maddon PJ, Koup RA, Moore JP, Paxton WA (1996) HIV-1 entry into CD4 cells is mediated by the chemokine receptor CC-CKR-5. Nature 381:667

40. Fang G, Burger H, Grimson R, Tropper P, Nachman S, Mayers D, Weislow O, Moore R, Reyelt C, Hutcheon N, Baker D, Weiser B (1995) Maternal plasma human immunodeficiency virus type 1 RNA level: a determinant and projected threshold for mother-to-child transmission. Proc Natl Acad Sci USA 92:12100

41. Feng Y, Broder CC, Kennedy PE, Berger EA (1996) HIV-1 entry cofactor: functional cDNA cloning of a seven-transmembrane G protein-coupled receptor. Science 272:872

42. Goedert JJ, Duliege A-M, Amos CI, Felton S, Biggar RJ (1991) High risk of HIV-1 infection for first-born twins. Lancet 338:1471

43. Horuk R (1994) Molecular properties of the chemokine receptor family. Trends Pharmacol Sci 15:159

44. Imagawa D, Detels R (1991) HIV-1 seronegative homosexual men. N Engl J Med 325:1250

45. Imagawa DT, Lee MH, Wolinsky SM, Sano K, Morales F, Kwok S, Sninsky JJ, Nishanian PG, Giorgi J, Fahey JL, Detels R (1989) Human immunodeficiency virus type 1 infection in homosexual men who remain seronegative for prolonged periods. N Engl J Med 320:1458

46. Jehuda-Cohen T, Slade B, Powell J, Villinger F, De B, Folks T, McClure H, Sell K, Ahmed-Ansari A (1990) Polyclonal B cell activation reveals antibodies against HIV-1 in HIV-1 seronegative individuals. Proc Natl Acad Sci USA 87:3972

47. Just J, Louie L, Abrams E, Nicholas SW, Wara D, Stein Z, King MC (1992) Genetic risk factors for perinatally acquired HIV-1 infection. Paediatr Perinat Epidemiol 6:215

48. Kaslow RA, Duquesnoy R, VanRaden M, Kingsley L, Marrari M, Friedman H, Su S, Saah AJ, Detels R, Phair J (1990) A1, Cw7, B8, DR3 HLA antigen combination associated with rapid decline of T helper lymphocytes in HIV-1 infection. A report from the Multicenter AIDS Cohort Study. Lancet 335:927

49. Kelker HC, Seidlin M, Vogler M, Valentine FT (1992) Lymphocytes from some long-term seronegative heterosexual partners of HIV infected individuals proliferate in response to HIV antigens. AIDS Res Human Retroviruses 8:1355
50. Kilpatrick DC, Hague RA, Yap PL, Mok JY (1991) HLA antigen frequencies in children born to HIV-infected mothers. Dis Markers 9:21
51. Kingsley LA, Detels R, Kaslow R, Polk BF, Rinaldo CRJ, Chmiel J, Detre K, Kelsey SF, Odaka N, Ostrow D, VanRaden M, Visscher B (1987) Risk factors for seroconversion to human immunodeficiency virus among male homosexuals. Lancet I:345
52. Klein MR, Keet IP, D'Amaro J, Bende RJ, Hekman A, Mesman B, Koot M, Waal LP de, Coutinho RA, Miedema F (1994) Associations between HLA frequencies and pathogenic features of human immunodeficinecy virus type 1 infection in seroconverters from Amsterdam cohort of homosexual men. J Infect Dis 169:1244
53. Korber BT, Learn G, Mullins JI, Hahn BH, Wolinsky S (1995) Protecting HIV databases. Nature 378:242
54. Koup RA, Ho DD (1991) Immunosilent HIV-1 infection: intrigue continues. J Acquir Immune Defic Syndr 5:1263
55. Koup R, Cao Y, Ho DD, Krogstad PA, Chen ISY, Korber BT, Wolinsky SM, Mullins J, Walker BD, Ammann A, The Ariel Project Cohort Group (1996) Lack of a maternal viral threshold for vertical transmission of HIV-1. Abstracts of the 3rd Conference on Retroviruses and Opportunistic Infections. (Infectious Diseases Society of America for the Foundation for Retrovirology and Human Health) abstr. no. LB2
56. Krieger JN, Coombs RW, Collier AC, Ho DD, Ross SO, Zeh JE, Corey L (1995) Intermittent shedding of human immunodeficiency virus in semen: implications for sexual transmission. J Urol 154:1035
57. Landesman SH, Kalish LA, Burns DN, Minkoff H, Fox HE, Zorrilla C, Garcia P, Fowler MG, Mofenson L, Tuomala R (1996) Obstetrical factors and the transmission of human immunodeficiency virus type 1 from mother to child. The Women and Infants Transmission Study. N Engl J Med 334:1617
58. Langlade-Demoyen P, Ngo-Giang-Huong N, Ferchal F, Oksenhendler E (1994) Human immunodeficiency virus (HIV) nef-specific cytotoxic T lymphocytes in noninfected heterosexual contact of HIV-infected patients. J Clin Invest 93:1293
59. Lederman MM, Jackson BJ, Kroner BL, White GCI, Eyster ME, Aledort LM, Hilgartner MW, Kessler CM, Cohen AR, Kiger KP, Goedert JJ (1995) Human immunodeficiency virus (HIV) type 1 infection status and in vitro susceptibility to HIV infection among high-risk HIV-1-seronegative hemophilicas. J Infect Dis 172:228
60. Lehner T, Wang Y, Cranage M, Bergmeier LA, Mitchell E, Tao L, Hall G, Dennis M, Cook N, Brookes R, Klavinskis L, Jones I, Doyle C, Ward R (1996) Protective mucosal immunity elicited by targeted iliac lymph node immunization with a subunit SIV enevelope and core vaccine in macaques. Nature Med 2:767
61. Levy JA (1993) HIV pathogenesis and long-term survival. J Acquir Immune Defic Syndr 7:1401
62. Levy JA (1993) Pathogenesis of human immunodeficiency virus infection. Microbiol Rev 57:183
63. Levy JA, Mackewicz CE, Barker E (1996) Controlling HIV pathogenesis: the role of the noncytotoxic anti-HIV response of CD8+ T cells. Immunol Today 17:217
64. Liu R, Paxton WA, Choe S, Ceradini D, Martin SR, Horuk R, MacDonald ME, Stuhlmann H, Koup RA, Landau NR (1996) Homozygous defect in HIV-1 coreceptor accounts for resistance of some multiply-exposed individuals to HIV-1 infection. Cell (in press)
65. Liuzzi G, Bagnarelli P, Chirianni A, Clementi M, Nappa S, Tullio Cataldo P, Valenza A, Piazza M (1995) Quantitation of HIV-1 genome copy number in semen and saliva. J Acquir Immune Defic Syndr 9:651
66. Lohman BL, Miller CJ, McChesney MB (1995) Antiviral cytotoxic T lymphocytes in vaginal mucosa of simian immunodeficiency virus-infected rhesus macaques. J Immunol 12:5855
67. Ludlam CA, Tucker J, Steel CM, Tedder RS, Cheingsong-Popov R, Weiss RA, McClelland DBL, Philip I, Prescott RJ (1985) HTLV-III infection in seronegative heamophiliacs after transfusion of Factor VIII. Lancet II:233
68. Lukacher AE, Braciale VL, Braciale TJ (1984) In vivo effector function of influenza virus-specific cytotoxic T lymphocyte clones is highly specific. J Exp Med 160:814
69. Mackewicz C, Levy JA (1992) CD8+ cell anti-HIV activity: nonlytic suppression of virus replication. J Acquir Immune Defic Syndr Res Hum Retroviruses 8:1039

70. Maggi E, Mazzetti M, Ravina A, Annunziato F, Carli M de, Piccinni MP, Manetti R, Carbonari M, Pesce AM, DelPrete G, Romagnani S (1994) Ability of HIV to promote a TH1 to TH0 shift and to replicate preferentially in TH2 and TH0 cells. Science 265:244

71. Marcus R (1988) Surveillance of health care workers exposed to blood from patients infected with HIV. N Engl J Med 319:1118

72. Mayaux MJ, Blanche S, Rouzioux C, Le Chenadec J, Chambrin V, Firtion G, Allemon MC, Vilmer E, Vigneron NC, Tricoire J (1995) Maternal factors associated with prenatal HIV-1 transmission: the French Cohort Study. J Acquir Immune Defic Synd Hum Retrovirology 8:188

73. McMichael A, Koup R, Ammann A (1996) Transient HIV infection in infants. N Engl J Med 334:801

74. Moses S, Plummer FA, Bradley J, Ndinya-Achola JO, Nagelkerke NJD, Ronald AR (1994) The association between lack of male circumcision and risk for HIV infection: A review of epidemiological data. Sex Transm Dis 21(4):201

75. Mosmann TR, Cherwinski H, Bond MW, Giedlin MA, Coffman RL (1986) Two types of murine helper T cell clone I. Definition according to profiles of lymphokine activities and secreted proteins. J Immunol 136:2348

76. O'Brien TR, Busch MP, Donegan E, Ward JW, Wong L, Samson SM, Perkins HA, Altman R, Stoneburner RL, Holmberg SD (1994) Heterosexual transmission of human immunodeficiency virus type 1 from transfusion recipients to their sex partners. J Acquir Immune Defic Syndr Hum Retrovirology 7:705

77. Ometto L, Zanotto C, Maccabruni A, Caselli D, Truscia D, Giaquinto C, Ruga E, Chieco-Bianchi L, De Rossi A (1995) Viral phenotype and host cell susceptibility to HIV-1 infection as risk factors for mother-to-child HIV-1 transmission. J Acquir Immune Defic Syndr 9:427

78. Pan L-Z, Sheppard HW, Winkelstein W, Levy JA (1991) Lack of detection of HIV in persistently seronegative homosexual men with high or medium risks for infection. J Infect Dis 164:962

79. Paxton WA, Martin SR, Tse D, O'Brien TR, Skurnick J, VanDevanter NL, Padian N, Braun JF, Kotler DP, Wolinsky SM, Koup RA (1996) Relative resistance to HIV-1 infection of CD4 lymphocytes from persons who remain uninfected despite multiple high-risk sexual exposures. Nature Med 2:412

80. Pinto LA, Sullivan J, Berzofsky JA, Clerici M, Kessler HA, Landay AL, Shearer GM (1995) Env specific cytotoxic T lymphocyte responses in HIV-seronegative health care workers occupationally exposed to HIV contaminated body fluids. J Clin Invest 96:867

81. Plourde PJ, Pepin J, Agoki E, Ronald AR, Ombette J, Tyndall M, Cheang M, Ndinya-Achola JO, D'Costa LJ, Plummer FA (1994) Human immunodeficiency virus type 1 seroconversion in women with gential ulcers. J Infect Dis 170:313

82. Plummer FA, Simonsen JN, Cameron DW, Ndinya-Achola JO, Kreiss JK, Gakinya MN, Waiyaki P, Cheang M, Piot P, Ronald AR, Ngugi EN (1991) Cofactors in male-female sexual transmission of human immunodeficiency virus type 1. J Infect Dis 163:233

83. Prevots DR, Ancelle-Park RA, Neal JJ, Remis RS (1994) The epidemiology of hetersexually acquired HIV infection and AIDS in western industrialized countries. J Acquir Immune Defic Syndr 8:S109

84. Rasheed S, Li Z, Xu D (1995) Human immunodeficiency virus load. Quantitative assessment in semen from seropositive individuals and in spiked seminal plasma. J Reprod Med 40:747

85. Roos MTL, Lange JMA, Goede REY de, Coutinho RA, Schellekens PTA, Miedema F, Tersmette M (1992) Viral phenotype and immune response in primary human immunodeficiency virus type 1 infection. J Infect Dis 165:427

86. Roques PA, Gras G, Parnet-Mathieu F, Mabondzo AM, Tranchot-Diallo J, Herve F, LasFargues G, Courpotin C, Dormont D (1995) Clearance of HIV infection in 12 perinatally infected children: clinical, virological and immunological data. J Acquir Immune Defic Syndr 9:F19

87. Rowland-Jones SL, Nixon DF, Gotch F, Hallam N, Froebel K, Aldhous MC, Ariyoshi K, Kroll JS, McMichael A (1993) HIV-specific cytotoxic T cell activity in an HIV-exposed but uninfected infant. Lancet 341:860

88. Rowland-Jones S, Sutton J, Ariyoshi K, Dong T, Gotch F, McAdam S, Whitby D, Sabally S, Gallimore A, Corrah T, Takiguchi M, Schultz T, McMichael A, Whittle H (1995) HIV-specific cytotoxic T cells in HIV-exposed but uninfected Gambian women. Nature Med 1:59

89. Salgame P, Abrams JS, Clayberger C, Goldstein H, Convit J, Modlin RL, Bloom BR (1991) Differing lymphokine profiles of functional subsets of human CD4 and CD8 T cell clones. Science 254:279

90. Salvato MS, Emau P, Malkovsky M, Schultz KT, Johnson E, Pauza CD (1994) Cellular immune responses in rhesus macaques infected rectally with low dose simian immunodeficiency virus. J Med Primatol 23:125

91. Schwartz RH (1985) T-lymphocyte recognition of antigen in association with gene products of the major histocompatibility complex. Annu Rev Immunol 3:237
92. Sethi KK, Omata Y, Schneweis KE (1983) Protection of mice from fatal herpes simplex virus type 1 infection by adoptive transfer of cloned virus-specific and H-2-restricted cytotoxic T lymphocytes. J Gen Virol 64:443
93. Simonsen JN, Cameron DW, Gakinya MN, Ndinya-Achola JO, D'Costa LJ, Karasira P, Cheang M, Ronald AR, Piot P, Plummer FA (1988) Human immunodeficiency virus infection among men with sexually transmitted diseases. N Engl J Med 319:274
94. Sperling RS, Shapiro DE, Coombs R, Todd J, McSherry G, Connor EM, Balsley J, Group AP0S (1996) Maternal plasma HIV-RNA and the success of zidovudine (ZDV) in the prevention of mother-child-transmission. Abstracts of the 3rd Conference on Retroviruses and Opportunistic Infections. (Infectious Diseases Society of America for the Foundation for Retrovirology and Human Health) abstr. no. LB1
95. Spira AI, Ho DD (1995) Effect of different donor cells on human immunodeficiency virus type 1 replication and selection in vitro. J Virol 69:422
96. Spira AI, Marx PA, Patterson BK, Mahoney J, Koup RA, Wolinsky SM, Ho DD (1996) Cellular targets of infection and route of viral dissemination following an intravaginal inoculation of SIV into rhesus macaques. J Exp Med 183:215
97. Steel CM, Ludlam CA, Beatson D, Peutherer JF, Cuthbert RJ, Simmonds P, Morrison H, Jones M (1988) HLA haplotype A1 B8 DR3 as a risk factor for HIV-related disease. Lancet I:1185
98. Stefano KA, Collman R, Kolson D, Hoxie J, Nathanson N, Gonzalez-Scarano F (1993) Replication of a macrophage-tropic strain of human immunodeficiency virus type 1 (HIV-1) in a hybrid cell line, CEMx174, suggests that cellular accessory molecules are required for HIV-1 entry. J Virol 67:6707
99. Stott J, Kitchin P, Page M, Flanagan B, Taffs L, Chan W, Mills K, Silvera P, Rodgers A (1991) Anti-cell antibody in macaques. Nature 353:393
100. Study, European Collaborative (1991) Risk factors for mother-to-child transmission of HIV-1. Lancet 339:1007
101. Taylor R (1994) Quiet clues to HIV-1 immunity: do some people resist infection? J NIH Res 6:29
102. Vyakaram A, Matear PM, Martin SJ, Wagstaff M (1995) Th1 cells specific for HIV-1 gag p24 are less efficient than Th0 cells in supporting HIV replication, and inhibit virus replication in Th0 cells. Immunology 86:85
103. Wainberg MA, Blain N, Fitz-Gibbon L (1987) Differential susceptibility of human lymphocyte cultures to infection by HIV. Clin Exp Immunol 1987:136
104. Walker CM, Moody DJ, Stites DP, Levy JA (1986) CD8$^+$ lymphocytes can control HIV infection in vitro by suppressing virus replication. Science 234:1563
105. Ward JW, Bush TJ, Perkins HA, Lieb LE, Allen JR, Goldfinger D, Samson SM, Pepkowitz SH, Fernando LP, Holland PV (1989) The natural history of transfusion-associated infection with human immunodeficiency virus. Factors influencing the rate of progression to disease. N Engl J Med 321:947
106. Williams LM, Cloyd MW (1991) Polymorphic human gene(s) determines differential susceptibility of CD4 lymphocytes to infection by certain HIV-1 isolates. Virology 184:723
107. Wolinsky SM, Wike CM, Korber BT, Hutto C, Parks WP, Rosenblum LL, Kunstman KJ, Furtado MR, Munoz JL (1992) Selective transmission of human immunodeficiency virus type-1 variants from mothers to infants. Science 255:1134
108. Yap KL, Ada GL (1978) The recovery of mice from influenza A infection: adoptive transfer of immunity with influenza virus-specific cytotoxic T lymphocytes recognizing a common virion antigen. Scand J Immunol 8:413
109. Zhang LQ, MacKenzie P, Cleland A, Holmes EC, Leigh Brown AJ, Simmonds P (1993) Selection for specific sequences in the external envelope protein of human immunodeficiency virus type 1 upon primary infection. J Virol 67:3345
110. Zhu T, Mo H, Wang N, Nam DS, Cao Y, Koup RA, Ho DD (1993) Genotypic and phenotypic characterization of HIV-1 in patients with primary infection. Science 261:1179
111. Zhu T, Wang N, Carr A, Nam DS, Moor-Jankowski R, Cooper DA, Ho DD (1996) Genetic characterization of human immunodeficiency virus type 1 in blood and genital secretions: evidence for viral compartmentalization and selection during sexual transmission. J Virol 70:3098

HIV-1-specific cytotoxic T lymphocytes and the control of HIV-1 replication

Christian Jassoy[1], Bruce D. Walker[2]

[1] Institute for Virology and Immunobiology, Julius-Maximilians University, Würzburg, Germany
[2] AIDS Research Center, Massachusetts General Hospital, Harvard Medical School, Fruit Street, Boston, MA 02114, USA

Introduction

In the 10 years since the identification of HIV-1-specific cytotoxic T lymphocytes (CTL) in infected persons, this cellular immune response has been investigated in more depth than in any other human viral infection. Despite substantial advances in understanding many features of this arm of the host defense, fundamental issues regarding the role of CTL in protecting from disease progression remain undefined, and the failure of CTL to effectively compete with the virus over the course of infection is unexplained. Recent advances from numerous laboratories are now beginning to shed light on these issues, and form the basis for the generation of new hypotheses.

CTL as an antiviral host defense mechanism

Viruses are intracellular pathogens, the replicative cycle of which includes a phase of potentially unique vulnerability to CTL. Following infection, enveloped viruses become uncoated, and the viral genome serves as the template for synthesis of new viral proteins. As proteins are produced for packaging into new virions, a competing process of cytoplasmic proteolysis also occurs. These processed proteins are transported to the endoplasmic reticulum where they form a complex with developing major histocompatibility complex (MHC) class I molecules, and are subsequently presented at the cell surface as a trimolecular complex consisting of peptide, class I molecule and β2-microglobulin. If CTL recognition of complex occurs before infectious viral progeny are produced, then host cell death leads to death of the virus. An effective CTL response should theoretically lead to elimination of infectious virus if the viral genomic material has not yet been packaged into the protective envelope derived from the host cell membrane. Early studies with vaccinia virus-infected cells demonstrated that immune spleen cells could decrease viral progeny production in vitro, providing

Correspondence to: C. Jassoy

experimental support for the hypothesis that CTL could kill virus-infected cells before the production of infectious progeny virus [101].

Experimental data in animals, and more recent data in humans have established that CTL can mediate a potent antiviral effect. In animal models, transfer of CTL at the time of virus challenge as well as after the establishment of productive infection have been shown to have protective effects (reviewed in [60]). Adoptive transfer of virus-specific CTL performed in a murine model of influenza virus infection demonstrated protection against a normally lethal virus inoculum delivered 24 h earlier [99]. Similar results were observed in murine herpes simplex virus (HSV) infection, where elevated levels of interferon-γ (IFN-γ) suggested that cytokine release by CTL might contribute to the antiviral effect [86]. The most extensively studied animal model of CTL is murine lymphocytic choriomeningitis virus (LCMV) infection, where kinetic studies indicate that adoptive transfer of LCMV-specific CTL can totally clear infectious virus within 24 h [11]. It is in the LCMV model that the essential role of cell killing was defined by the demonstration that perforin-knockout mice are unable to clear LCMV infection in vivo [41], although additional studies have shown fas-fas ligand interactions to also contribute to cell killing [43, 54].

New data in humans also contribute evidence that CTL can mediate a protective effect. Early studies demonstrated correlations between CTL induction and recovery from influenza [61] and cytomegalovirus (CMV) [78] infection, and recent human studies of CMV-specific CTL responses following bone marrow transplantation have extended these observations. Adoptive transfer of donor CMV-specific CTL following bone marrow transplant effectively reconstituted cellular immunity against CMV, and none of the 14 recipients studied developed CMV viremia or disease [95]. These results have been further extended in human Epstein-Barr virus (EBV) infection by the demonstration that adoptively transferred EBV-specific CTL not only restore EBV-specific cellular immunity but that these cells can still respond to in vivo or ex vivo viral challenge 18 months later [32]. Collectively, these data provide strong evidence that virus-specific CTL are an important and potentially effective host immune response.

CTL in HIV-1 infection

In 1987 HIV-specific CTL activity was reported in infected individuals using freshly isolated mononuclear cells derived from the peripheral blood (PBMC) [91] and from bronchoalveolar lavage [76]. This cytotoxic activity was detected without prior in vitro stimulation of the cells, an observation that was unprecedented because of the usual need for initial rounds of in vitro stimulation for the detection of virus-specific CTL responses in other viral infections. In addition, the detection of this vigorous cellular immune response was unexpected in HIV infection given the fact that the disease is characterized by progressive and ultimately profound immunosuppression [72]. Perhaps one of the most surprising findings regarding the in vivo-activated CTL response is that it can be maintained at high levels and can be broadly directed in some long-term non-progressors in whom the viral load is below the limit of detection (< 200 RNA molecules/ml plasma), indicating that strong CTL responses may not require high viral loads to persist in vivo [28, 29].

Since those initial descriptions, studies from numerous laboratories have contributed to a more comprehensive understanding of the targets of the CTL response in infected persons. Using recombinant vaccinia viruses encoding HIV structural and regulatory proteins, it has been observed that the CTL response can be directed at multiple proteins in a single individual, with as many as 14 different epitopes having been described to be targeted in a single individual [39]. The most frequently recognized (but also most frequently studied) proteins are the Gag, polymerase, Env and Nef proteins (reviewed in [60]). CTL responses against the regulatory proteins Vif, Tat, Rev, intergrase, and proteinase have also been detected, but may be present at a lower frequency [52, 83]. The use of target cells incubated with synthetic HIV-1 peptides has resulted in the identification of over three dozen CTL epitopes and their restricting class I antigens (reviewed in [9, 60]). These epitopes conform to the expected motif predictions based on elution of peptides from class-I molecules, which typically range from eight to ten amino acids in length [19, 20], although longer epitopes have been described.

The vigor of the HIV-specific CTL response in fresh peripheral blood from infected individuals is mirrored by the high precursor frequency of CTL [13, 50]. For example, Gag-specific CTL precursors have been documented at frequencies of up to 1 per 300 lymphocytes in long-term asymptomatic persons, and have been observed to decline with disease progression [48]. Similarly, envelope-specific CTL have been reported at frequencies up to 1 per 1000 PBMC [44]. Our own studies have detected CTL precursors specific for a single epitope at frequencies of up to 1 per 500 cells (unpublished data), and T cell receptor (TCR) analysis has indicated not only that these cells can be oligoclonal but that a single clone can persist in vivo for over 4 years ([44] and unpublished data). These numbers may actually underestimate the true frequency of CTL, since precursor frequency analysis may not detect the already activated fraction of CTL [24]. Using an oligonucleotide probe to the CDR3 region of the TCR, it has been shown that a single CTL clone can comprise up to 1% of the T cell transcripts in peripheral blood [67]. Our own studies using TCR analysis have shown that a single CTL clone can constitute 3% or more of the circulating CD8 cell population during chronic stable infection (unpublished data).

HIV-1-specific CTL have been detected not only in peripheral blood and lung, but also in other body fluids and tissues of infected individuals, and it has been suggested that CTL may contribute to disease pathogenesis in certain tissues [102]. For example, examination of the cerebrospinal fluid (CSF) of individuals with HIV-associated dementia revealed CTL activity which was broadly directed at epitopes in the HIV Gag, RT, Env, and Nef proteins [36, 37, 77] and a similar broadly directed CTL response was recently observed in the CSF and brain tissue of simian immunodeficiency virus (SIV)-infected rhesus macaques [89]. The frequency with which CTL were isolated and the observation that CTL derived from the CSF and brain often recognized viral proteins different from those identified in the blood may suggest differences in the CTL response in these compartments [89]. Immunohistologic examinations demonstrated that lymphocytic meningitis characterized by CD8$^+$ T cell infiltrates in leptomeninges and perivascular spaces are common within the brain in presymptomatic stages of HIV infection. The presence of CD8$^+$ T cells in vascular inflammation suggests that these cells may participate in the immunologic control of viral replication in the central nervous system (reviewed in: [25]), whereas analogies to LCMV infection suggest that cytokines released by these activated CTL may contribute to the neuropathologic changes associated with HIV infection [38].

Other tissues have also been shown to contain CTL. A skin rash frequently occurs as a primary clinical manifestation of HIV and SIV infection, and the exanthem is accompanied by infiltration of CD8$^+$ T lymphocytes in the dermis and epidermis and variable epidermal injury [82]. Antigen-specific CD8$^+$ CTL have been detected in the inflamed skin of SIV-infected rhesus macaques at the time of primary infection, suggesting that the presence of SIV-specific CTL activity may be linked to the development of the skin erythema [96]. Furthermore, HIV- and SIV-specific CD8$^+$ CTL responses have been detected in lymphoid tissue [26, 81] and the spleen [26] of infected individuals and monkeys. Histologic analyses provide additional support for the presence and activity of CTL in lymphatic tissue. The numbers of CD8$^+$ T lymphocytes were dramatically increased in lymph nodes of HIV-infected individuals with lymphadenopathy, primarily due to an increase of the memory T cell subtype [79]. Evidence that a large fraction of these cells are cytotoxic cells was obtained by in situ hybridization of the enzyme serine esterase B which is a component of cytoplasmic granules of CTL and demonstrated the presence of cytolytic cells within follicles of hyperplastic lymph nodes of HIV-infected individuals [18]. Similarly, immunostaining of cytotoxic granules with the anti-TIA monoclonal antibody indicated the existence of large numbers of cytotoxic CD8$^+$ T lymphocytes in germinal centers of hyperplastic lymphoid follicles. However, a marked loss of CD8$^+$ TIA$^+$ cells was observed in lymphocyte-depleted lymph nodes of patients with AIDS [87].

Besides HIV-specific CD8$^+$ CTL, CD4$^+$ envelope glycoprotein-specific CTL have been derived from the peripheral blood of vaccinated seronegative individuals and the culture of a CD4$^+$ Gag-specific CTL line has been described. Their function and significance have recently been discussed elsewhere [35] and are not considered in this review.

Can CTL control virus replication?

The ability of CTL to inhibit viral replication requires that the host cell be lysed before the full yield of infectious virus is produced. An antiviral effect by CTL should be readily achieved for non-cytopathic viruses, since the infected cell may otherwise persist and release infectious virions for extended periods of time. In contrast, it has been postulated that lysis of infected cells by CTL occurs too late in the life cycle of cytopathic viruses for lysis to be effective, because a maximal yield of infectious virus may already have been assembled and be released on lysis of the cell [42]. Such a hypothesis is supported by experimental data indicating that perforin-dependent mechanisms are not a major component of protection in infections with cytopathic viruses, such as vaccinia or vesicular stomatitis virus [43], in which cytokines such as IFN released by CTL may represent an important soluble mediator of viral suppression [68].

Recent dynamic studies of HIV pathogenesis indicate that the average HIV life cycle from infection of one cell to production of viral progeny and subsequent new rounds of infection is slightly greater than 2 days [74] and, thus, the window of opportunity for antiviral CTL is very short. Most studies of CTL function have measured lysis of chromium-labeled target cells infected with vaccinia viruses expressing recombinant viral proteins or labeled with synthetic peptides, and thus have not defined when an infected CD4 cell becomes susceptible to CTL-mediated lysis. Kinetic studies using synchronous HIV infection of susceptible CD4 cells are now beginning to shed light on this issue [98]. In these studies HIV susceptible CD4$^+$ cell lines were infected at a high multiplicity of infection, leading to detection of intracellular p24 antigen expression by 1–2 days after infection, and resulting in greater than 98% of cells positive for HIV p24 by 3–4 days. Recognition of infected cells by HIV-specific CTL clones closely paralleled intracellular p24 antigen expression, and preceded peak virion production. Thus, infected cells appear to be recognized very early in the virus life cycle, at least if CTL are present in the local microenvironment of the infected CD4 cells. These same studies demonstrated that HIV-1 infection was associated with a 50% decrease in HLA class I expression, but this decrease was not associated with a negative effect on lysis by CTL. Whether these decreases in class I expression are associated with a decreased ability of CTL to inhibit virus replication still needs to be determined, but these studies indicate that infected cells can be recognized early in the life cycle, an essential characteristic if CTL are to mediate an antiviral effect.

CTL and suppression of HIV replication in vitro

In HIV-infected individuals, continued virus replication takes place in the face of a vigorous cellular immune response. The ability of CTL to recognize infected cells early in the virus life cycle suggests that these cells may be able to effectively inhibit virus replication, yet definitive studies which resolve this issue are lacking. Nevertheless, several lines of evidence indicate that cellular immune responses are active against viral spread in vivo. In vitro studies demonstrate that removal of CD8$^+$ T cells from PBMC of seropositive asymptomatic individuals facilitates isolation of HIV from CD4 cells when they are stimulated in vitro with mitogen [92]. CD8$^+$ T cells from these individuals inhibit virus replication when added both at the initiation of virus infection and after a productive viral infection has been established. Whether suppression involves cytolysis of infected cells remains controversial. One study demonstrated that virus-containing cells were not eliminated from the culture [93]. In addition, virus suppression was not HLA restricted and was cross-reactive against several HIV-1, HIV-2, and SIV isolates [94]. In contrast, another study demonstrated that the effector cells had phenotypic characteristics consistent with CTL [88]. CD8$^+$ T cells from uninfected donors have been shown to be less inhibitory in some studies, although other studies have clearly demonstrated an ability of CD8 cells from uninfected persons to inhibit replication [5, 10]. CD8 cells from both infected and uninfected persons have recently been shown to inhibit HIV replication in an "endogenous system", in which mixtures of CD4 cells and dendritic cells from infected persons are used in the assay system. In contrast, only CD8 cells from infected persons inhibit replication when an acute infection system is used, in which CD4 cell/dendritic cell mixtures from uninfected persons are infected in vitro [5].

   The extent of antiviral activity may correlate with the clinical status of the donor and range from asymptomatic individuals, who exhibit strong CD8$^+$ T cell anti-HIV activity, to patients with AIDS, who show the lowest degree of activity [12, 55], although a subpopulation of infected individuals with very high CD4$^+$ T cell numbers and low virus burden may not secrete the HIV-suppressing factor spontaneously [22]. In addition, non-cytolytic anti-HIV activity was detectable in the plasma of HIV-infected individuals several months before neutralizing antibodies were found [56]. The antiviral suppressive activity was primarily exhibited by CD28$^+$, HLA-DR$^+$, CD8$^+$ T cells and partly mediated by a soluble factor, although optimal activity may have required cell-cell contact. The CD8$^+$ T cell antiviral factor arrested virus replication at the transcriptional level [14, 57], is soluble, heat and pH stable and smaller than 30 kDa

[53]. The factor is reportedly none of the known cytokines including interleukins (IL), IFN and tumor necrosis factors (TNF) (reviewed in [53]). Recent conflicting reports suggest that the combination of RANTES, MIP-1α and MIP-1β [16] or IL-16 [3] may be the elusive suppressive factor. It is not clear at this point whether one or several factors may have to act synergistically and which stimulus may trigger its or their release. The complexity of the situation is further underscored by the demonstration that the soluble factors released by CD8 cells can enhance HIV replication in certain experimental situations [27]. Since soluble anti-HIV activity secreted by CD8$^+$ T cells from seronegative individuals has also been described [5, 10], it raises the likelihood that factor-mediated soluble suppression may be intrinsic to activated CD8$^+$ cells.

In most of the studies reporting soluble antiviral activity derived from CD8$^+$ T cells, the character and function of the T cells involved in mediating this effect have not been further identified, and it remains to be clarified whether all or only a subset of CD8$^+$ T cells are able to release the antiviral factor(s). A number of cytokines and chemokines have been demonstrated to be released by antiviral CTL upon stimulation with the cognate epitope, and the high frequency of HIV-specific CTL in infected persons certainly raises the possibility that these cells may contribute to the observed antiviral effects of CD8 cells. Examination of HIV-specific CD8$^+$ CTL clones derived from the peripheral blood and from the CSF of HIV-infected individuals demonstrated that after contact with the relevant target, CTL released IFN-γ, TNF-α, TNF-β [37] granulocyte/macrophage-colony-stimulating factor and variable amounts of IL-2, IL-3, and IL-4 in an HLA-restricted fashion [77]. In addition, our unpublished data indicate that both HIV- and hepatitis C virus-specific CTL clones release the chemokines RANTES, MIP-1α and MIP-1β in an HLA-restricted epitope-specific fashion. Experiments performed in the SIV system point to a specific subset of CD8$^+$ T cells that exhibited the capacity to inhibit virus replication by demonstrating that the CD8$^+$ T cells involved had the characteristics of CTL [88]. In these studies, CD8$^+$ T cells blocked virus replication in autologous but not in HLA-mismatched cells. In addition, physical contact was required since virus replication was blocked by antibodies against CD8 and lymphocyte function-associated antigen-1 [45, 46, 88]. Nevertheless, the involvement of CTL in virus suppression remains controversial.

Protection from disease progression in viral infections may be mediated by direct cytotoxicity or by cytokines released by the CTL, and the relative contributions of these effector mechanisms may depend on the virus and animal system under study [58, 80]. The contribution of direct cytotoxic activity and cytokines released by the CTL on HIV replication has been addressed experimentally using HIV-1 infected CD4$^+$ cell lines as target cells [97]. When H9 cells are transfected with the HLA-B14 molecule, virus replication can be inhibited by 10^5-fold by HLA B14-restricted CTL clones, when compared to the level of replication seen in the absence of added clone or in the absence of the restricting B14 molecule. This recognition leads to the release of soluble inhibitors of HIV replication which have the characteristics of the CD8 antiviral factor reported by Levy and collaborators; however, the degree of inhibition achieved with the soluble factor is much less than that observed with direct HLA-matched cell contact. These data indicate that CTL inhibit HIV by both cytolytic and non-cytolytic mechanisms. The ability of CTL to produce soluble inhibitory factors when they encounter their target antigen may confer a benefit in the local microenvironment in vivo by decreasing infection by viruses which may already have been produced by the targeted cell. The functions of HIV-specific CTL and their action on viral replication are summarized in Fig. 1.

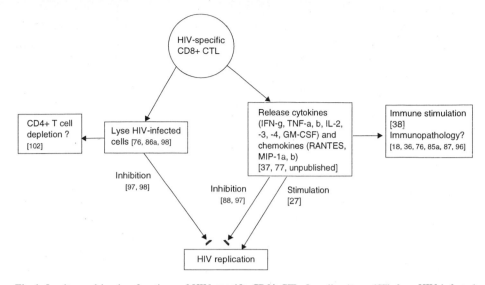

Fig. 1. In vitro and in vivo functions of HIV specific CD8[+] CTL. In cell culture, CTL lyse HIV-infected primary lymphocytes, macrophages and transformed lymphoblastoid cells. Moreover, CTL release a variety of cytokines upon contact with antigen-expressing cells. Both direct cell lysis and cytokines inhibit HIV replication in vitro. However, in particular circumstances, cytokines released by CTL may stimulate virus replication. It is still a matter of debate how these in vitro observations relate to the in vivo situation. Certainly, ongoing virus replication constitutes the basis for continuing activation and proliferation of HIV-specific CTL. A wealth of data indicate that CTL limit HIV replication in the infected individual. However, does killing of infected CD4[+] T cells by CD8[+] CTL cause CD4[+] T cell depletion? Similarly, do cytokines released by CTL contribute to immune stimulation and pathology in the affected tissues?

Potential mechanisms for HIV-1 persistence in the presence of CTL

Despite the presence of a vigorous CTL response, HIV is not eliminated and a productive chronic infection is established. The level of viremia following primary infection is a strong predictor of subsequent disease progression [63, 71, 84], and the appearance of HIV-specific CTL coincident with the drop in peak viremia suggests that CTL are at least partially effective in containing the virus [7, 51]. TCR analysis demonstrating restricted expansions of variable domain beta chain ($V\beta$) families which mediate HIV-1-specific cytotoxicity provides further compelling evidence that class I-restricted CTL are a component to the primary immune response to HIV infection [73]. However, the inability of the HIV-specific CTL response to eliminate virus remains unexplained. A number of hypotheses regarding potential mechanisms of HIV persistence have been proposed, including avoidance of immune surveillance as well as viral immunomodulatory effects. Experimental data are accruing which begin to support both of these mechanisms in HIV infection.

Viral escape from immune surveillance has been well demonstrated in murine models of virus infection. In vitro, low-dose infection of fibroblasts in the presence of CTL specific for a defined LCMV glycoprotein epitope has been shown to result in the emergence of escape viruses due to single point mutations, resulting in single amino acid changes. These mutations which result in non-recognition by the CTL were found to occur frequently [1]. In vivo, LCMV infection of mice transgenic for an LCMV-specific TCR resulted in selection for virus variants which were not recognized by the existing CTL response [75]. These studies examined a situation in that simultaneous mutations within all epitopes would not be likely. It has been shown that escape from some but not all epitopes confers an advantage to the virus [66], providing further support for the hypothesis that escape is an important mechanism of persistence.

Studies in HIV-infected persons have also identified sequence variation within CTL epitopes, although the overall contribution of CTL immune escape to disease progression remains unresolved. In persons with chronic infection, mutations within defined epitopes are commonly identified, but the effects of such variation on CTL recognition is complex. Mutations within important anchor residues have been shown to result in lack of peptide-HLA binding, thus rendering epitopes unrecognized [17]. However, mutations within residues involved more in interaction with the TCR may have modest or no effects on recognition by established CTL responses, and may also generate new immune responses. Detailed longitudinal studies have shown fluctuating mutations not seen by the CTL of a patient who progressed, whereas a dominant and sustained response to a single Gag epitope was observed in a person with non-progressing disease [70]. These limited studies need to be expanded to determine the frequency of such events. It is clear that allowable mutations are not a consistent finding in the setting of strong CTL pressure [15, 64, 69], leaving open not only the role of CTL pressure in driving HIV-1 evolution in vivo, but also the necessity of immune escape for disease progression. A recently proposed mathematical model attempted to define the interaction between CTL and dominant epitopes of genetically variable viruses [70]. This model suggests that antigenic variation can shift CTL responses from dominant to subdominant epitopes, with a resultant decrease in the ability of CTL to contain the virus.

In addition to sequence variation leading to MHC binding or lack of TCR recognition, another mechanism for immune escape by genetically variable viruses has been proposed. Termed antagonism, this process involves altered peptide ligands which bind to the MHC molecule and engage the TCR, but fail to induce a lethal hit by the CTL. Natural variants of hepatitis B virus [6] and HIV [49] have been shown to potently inhibit antiviral CTL, although the mechanism of this antagonism is not clear. All of these studies have relied on acute lysis of cells as a readout, using either peptide, recombinant vaccinia virus, or acute viral infection to express the altered peptide ligand [62]. Whether these alterations result in an inability of CTL to inhibit virus replication in vitro or in vivo remains to be determined. In our own studies, we have rarely been able to detect antagonism, suggesting that this mechanism may vary depending on the epitope, and restricting class I molecule, and/or the individual TCR.

Another mechanism of CTL immune evasion involves viral immunomodulatory molecules, an example of which is viral regulation of MHC-peptide complex expression. Cytopathic viruses such as vaccinia down-regulate MHC class I expression by shutting off host protein synthesis, but the effects of this down-regulation are likely to be minimal since the infected cells die and, therefore, do not serve as a persistent source of infectious virions. A more specific down-regulation of class I expression has been identified in HSV infection in which the protein product of the viral ICP47 gene causes retention of class I molecules in the endoplasmic reticulum [100]. ICP47 interferes with the function of the TAP1/TAP2 complex which transports cytosolic proteins to the endoplasmic reticulum [33]. Down-regulation of class I expression has also been shown for human CMV infection [4] and adenovirus infection [31]. The ability of HIV-1 to inhibit class I expression has been demonstrated in a number of studies, although the precise mechanism is not clear. One study showed a 12-fold decrease in the activity of a class I gene promoter by the Tat protein, but the biologic effect of this down-regulation has not been defined [34]. Another viral protein which has been postulated to affect immune clearance is the vpr gene, which induces a cell cycle arrest [30, 40, 47]. However, the demonstration that lysis by CTL was unimpaired by HIV infection of susceptible CD4 cells [98] raises further questions about the relevance of these effects in vivo.

In considering the issue of viral persistence in HIV-1 infection, one must also consider the unique features of this virus which are likely to contribute to disease pathogenesis. Because HIV-1 infects CD4$^+$ cells by virtue of specific binding to CD4 in addition to a second receptor [2, 21], these cells are rendered dysfunctional in the earliest stages of infection studied to date, and are progressively depleted over the course of the illness (reviewed in [65]). The most glaring defect in the immunologic repertoire in HIV infection compared to other viral infections is the lack of virus-specific CD4 helper cell function, and recent data from murine models of viral infections indicate a critical role for these cells. Although primary CTL responses can be generated in mice in the absence of CD4 cells, maintenance of CTL function during the chronic viral infection requires the presence of CD4 cells [59, 90]. In the absence of CD4 cells, mice challenged with LCMV have reduced CTL precursors as early as 30 days after immunization, and CD4-deficient mice are less efficiently protected from LCMV challenge. In HIV-1 infection, HIV-specific CD4 cells are rarely detected [85], and the progressive loss of CD4 cells may play a central role in the progressive loss of CTL function over the course of illness.

In addition to the loss of CD4 cells, HIV also infects a number of antigen-presenting cells (APC) such as monocyte-macrophages and Langerhans cells [23]. Infection of these cells may lead to immune elimination by CTL, or to direct cyto-pathic effects mediated by the virus. In mice, infection with an LCMV clone which causes widespread infection of APC results in CD8-mediated destruction of these cells, and contributes directly to immunosuppression [8]. Loss or dysfunction of APC in HIV infection may contribute to the observed inability of infected persons to maintain established CTL responses and/or to respond to new virus variants over time, and thus contribute to disease progression.

Conclusions

Despite more than a decade of vigorous worldwide research efforts, the correlates of protection from HIV-1 disease progression remain undefined. Numerous studies have confirmed the presence of a virus-specific CTL response in HIV-1 infection, the appearance of which correlates temporally with the decrease in primary viremia. These studies coupled with in vitro studies demonstrating the ability of CTL to inhibit HIV-1 replication, as well as the observed loss of HIV-1-specific CTL with disease progression all suggest that CTL help to control viral replication. The inability of CTL to actually clear the infection remains a central enigma, although the dysfunction and loss of CD4 helper cell function as well as defects in APC function induced by HIV infection may prove to be important contributors. Further studies which answer these questions are urgently needed to guide therapeutic and preventive interventions.

Acknowledgement. This work was supported by a grant from the Bundesministerium für Bildung, Wissenschaft, Forschung und Technologie (AIDS-Stipendienprogramm) and from the Deutsche Forschungsgemeinschaft, Bonn, Germany (C.J.); and by NIH grants R37 AI28568, RO1 AI30914, and the Ariel Project for the Prevention of HIV Transmission from Mother to Infant (B.D.W.).

References

1. Aebischer T, Moskophidis D, Rohrer UH, Zinkernagel RM, Hengartner H (1991) In vitro selection of lymphocytic choriomeningitis virus escape mutants by cytotoxic T lymphocytes. Proc Natl Acad Sci USA 88:11 047

2. Alkhatib G, Combadiere C, Broder CC, Feng Y, Kennedy PE, Murphy PM, Berger EA (1996) CC CKR5: a RANTES, MIP-1alpha, MIP-1beta receptor as a fusion cofactor for macrophage-tropic HIV-1. Science 272:1955

3. Baier M, Werner A, Bannert N, Metzner K, Kurth R (1995) HIV suppression by interleukin-16 (letter; comment). Nature 378:563

4. Banks TA, Rouse BT (1992) Herpes viruses – immune escape artists? (Review). Clin Infect Dis 14:933

5. Barker TD, Weissman D, Daucher JA, Roche KM, Fauci AS (1996) Identification of multiple and distinct CD8$^+$ T cell supressor activities. J Immunol 156:4476

6. Bertoletti A, Sette A, Chisari FV, Penna A, Levrero M, De-Carli M, Fiaccadori F, Ferrari C (1994) Natural variants of cytotoxic epitopes are T-cell receptor antagonists for antiviral cytotoxic T cells. Nature 369:407

7. Borrow P, Lewicki H, Hahn BH, Shaw GM, Oldstone MBA (1994) Virus-specific CD8$^+$ cytotoxic T-lymphocyte activity associated with control of viremia in primary human immunodeficiency virus type 1 infection. J Virol 68:6103

8. Borrow P, Evans CF, Oldstone MB (1995) Virus-induced immunosuppression: immune system-mediated destruction of virus-infected dendritic cells results in generalized immune suppression. J Virol 69:1059

9. Brander C, Walker BD (1995) The HLA-class I restricted CTL response in HIV-1 infection: identification of optimal epitopes. In: Koerber BTM, Brander C, Walker BD (eds) Theoretical biology and biophysics. HIV molecular immunology database. Los Alamos National Laboratory, Los Alamos

10. Brinchmann JE, Gaudernack G, Vartdal F (1990) CD8$^+$ T cells inhibit HIV replication in naturally infected CD4$^+$ T cells. Evidence for a soluble inhibitor. J Immunol 144:2961

11. Byrne JA, Oldstone MB (1984) Biology of cloned cytotoxic T lymphocytes specific for lymphocytic choriomeningitis virus: clearance of virus in vivo. J Virol 51:682

12. Cao Y, Qin L, Zhang L, Safrit S, Ho DD (1995) Virologic and immunologic characterization of long-term survivors of human immunodeficiency virus type 1 infection (see comments). N Engl J Med 332:201

13. Carmichael A, Jin X, Sissons P, Borysiewicz L (1993) Quantitative analysis of the human immunodeficiency virus type 1 (HIV-1)-specific cytotoxic T lymphocyte (CTL) response at different stages of HIV-1 infection: differential CTL responses to HIV-1 and Epstein-Barr virus in late disease. J Exp Med 177:249

14. Chen C-H, Weinhold K, Bartlett JA, Bolognesi DP, Greenberg ML (1993) CD8 T lymphocyte-mediated inhibition of HIV-1 long terminal repeat transcription: a novel antiviral mechanism. AIDS Res Hum Retroviruses 9:1079

15. Chen ZW, Shen L, Miller MD, Ghim SH, Hughes AL, Letvin NL (1992) Cytotoxic T lymphocytes do not appear to select for mutations in an immunodominant epitope of simian immunodeficiency virus gag. J Immunol 149:4060

16. Cocchi F, DeVico AL, Garzino-Demo A, Arya SK, Gallo RC, Lusso P (1995) Identification of RANTES, MIP-1 alpha, and MIP-1 beta as the major HIV-suppressive factors produced by CD8$^+$ cells. Science 270:1811

17. Couillin I, Culmann-Penciolelli B, Gomard E, Choppin J, Levy J-P, Guillet J-G, Saragosti S (1994) Impaired cytotoxic T lymphocyte recognition due to genetic variations in the main immunogenic region of the human immunodeficiency virus 1 NEF protein. J Exp Med 180:1129

18. Devergne O, Peuchmaur M, Crevon MC, Trapani JA, Maillot MC, Galanaud P, Emilie D (1991) Activation of cytotoxic cells in hyperplastic lymph nodes from HIV-infected patients. AIDS 5:1071

19. Falk K, Rotzschke O, Deres K, Metzger J, Jung G, Rammensee HG (1991) Identification of naturally processed viral nonapeptides allows their quantification in infected cells and suggests an allele-specific T cell epitope forecast. J Exp Med 174:425

20. Falk K, Rotzschke O, Stevanovic S, Jung G, Rammensee HG (1991) Allele-specific motifs revealed by sequencing of self-peptides eluted from MHC molecules. Nature 351:290

21. Feng Y, Broder CC, Kennedy PE, Berger EA (1996) HIV-1 entry cofactor: functional cDNA cloning of a seven-transmembrane, G protein-coupled receptor (see comments). Science 272:872

22. Ferbas J, Kaplan AH, Hausner MA, Hultin LE, Matud JL, Liu Z, Panicali DL, Nerng-Ho H, Detels R, Giorgi JV (1995) Virus burden in long-term survivors of human immunodeficiency virus (HIV) infection is a determinant of anti-HIV CD8$^+$ lymphocyte activity. J Infect Dis 172:329

23. Franker SS, Wenig BM, Burke AP, Mannan P, Thompson LDR, Abbondanzo SL, Nelson AM, Pope M, Steinman RM (1996) Replication of HIV-1 in dendritic cell-derived syncytia at the mucosal surface of the adenoid. Science 272:115

24. Gotch FM, Nixon DF, Alp N, McMichael AJ, Borysiewicz LK (1990) High frequency of memory and effector gag specific cytotoxic T lymphocytes in HIV seropositive individuals. Int Immunol 2:707

25. Gray F, Scaravilli F, Everall I, Chretien F, An S, Boche D, Adle-Biassette H, Wingertsmann L, Durigon M, Hurtrel B, Chiodi F, Bell J, Lantos P (1996) Neuropathology of early HIV-1 infection. Brain Pathol 6:1

26. Hadida F, Parrot A, Kieny MP, Sadat SB, Mayaud C, Debre P, Autran B (1992) Carboxyl-terminal and central regions of human immunodeficiency virus-1 NEF recognized by cytotoxic T lymphocytes from lymphoid organs. An in vitro limiting dilution analysis. J Clin Invest 89:53

27. Harrer T, Jassoy C, Harrer E, Johnson RP, Walker BD (1993) Induction of HIV-1 replication in a chronically infected T-cell line by cytotoxic T lymphocytes. J Acquir Immune Defic Syndr 6:865

28. Harrer T, Harrer E, Kalams S, Barbosa P, Trocha A, Johnson R, Elbeik T, Feinberg M, Buchbinder S, Walker B (1996) Cytotoxic T lymphocytes in asymptomatic long-term non-progressing HIV-1 infection: breadth and specificity of the response and relation to in vivo viral quasispecies in a person with prolonged infection and low viral load. J Immunol 156:2616

29. Harrer T, Harrer E, Kalams SA, Trocha A, Johnson RP, Elbeik T, Feinberg M, Cao H, Ho DD, Buchbinder S, Walker B (1996) Strong cytotoxic T cells and weak neutralizing antibodies in a subset of persons with long-term non-progressing HIV-1 infection. AIDS Res Hum Retro 12:585

30. Heinzinger NK, Bukinsky MI, Haggerty SA, Ragland AM, Kewalramani V, Lee MA, Gendelman HE, Ratner L, Stevenson M, Emerman M (1994) The Vpr protein of human immunodeficiency virus type 1 influences nuclear localization of viral nucleic acids in nondividing host cells. Proc Natl Acad Sci USA 91:7311

31. Hermiston TW, Tripp RA, Sparer T, Gooding LR, Wold WS (1993) Deletion mutation analysis of the adenovirus type 2 E3-gp19K protein: identification of sequences within the endoplasmic reticulum lumenal domain that are required for class I antigen binding and protection from adenovirus-specific cytotoxic T lymphocytes. J Virol 67:5289

32. Heslop HE, Ng CY, Li C, Smith CA, Loftin SK, Krance RA, Brenner MK, Rooney CM (1996) Long term restoration of immunity against Epstein-Barr virus infection by adoptive transfer of gene-modified virus-specific T lymphocytes. Nature Med 2:551

33. Hill A, Jugovic P, York I, Russ G, Bennink J, Yewdell J, Ploegh H, Johnson D (1995) Herpes simplex virus turns off the TAP to evade host immunity. Nature 375:411

34. Howcroft TK, Strebel K, Martin MA, Singer DS (1993) Repression of MHC class I gene promoter activity by two-exon Tat of HIV. Science 260:1320

35. Jassoy C, Walker B (1996) Cytotoxic T lymphocytes and their cytokines in human immunodeficiency virus infection. Crit Rev Oncogen (in press)

36. Jassoy C, Johnson RP, Navia BA, Worth J, Walker BD (1992) Detection of a vigorous HIV-1-specific cytotoxic T lymphocyte response in cerebrospinal fluid from infected persons with AIDS dementia complex. J Immunol 149:3113

37. Jassoy C, Harrer T, Rosenthal T, Navia BA, Worth J, Johnson RP, Walker BD (1993) Human immunodeficiency virus type 1-specific cytotoxic T lymphocytes release gamma interferon, tumor necrosis factor alpha (TNF-alpha), and TNF-beta when they encounter their target antigens. J Virol 67:2844

38. Jassoy C, Heinkelein M, Klinker H, Walker BD (1994) HIV type 1-specific cytotoxic T lymphocytes stimulate HLA class I and intercellular adhesion molecule type 1 expression and increase beta 2-microglobulin levels in vitro. AIDS Res Hum Retroviruses 10:1685

39. Johnson R, Walker B (1994) Cytotoxic T lymphocytes in HIV infection: Responses to structural proteins. Curr Top Microbiol Immunol 189:35–62
40. Jowett JB, Planelles V, Poon B, Shah NP, Chen ML, Chen IS (1995) The human immunodeficiency virus type 1 vpr gene arrests infected T cells in the G2 + M phase of the cell cycle. J Virol 69:6304
41. Kagi D, Ledermann B, Burki K, Seiler P, Odermatt B, Olsen KJ, Podack ER, Zinkernagel RM, Hengartner H (1994) Cytotoxicity mediated by T cells and natural killer cells is greatly impaired in perforin-deficient mice. Nature 369:31
42. Kagi D, Ledermann B, Burki K, Zinkernagel RM, Hengartner H (1995) Lymphocyte-mediated cytotoxicity in vitro and in vivo: mechanisms and significance (Review). Immunol Rev 146:95
43. Kagi D, Seiler P, Pavlovic J, Ledermann B, Burki K, Zinkernagel RM, Hengartner H (1995) The roles of perforin- and Fas-dependent cytotoxicity in protection against cytopathic and noncytopathic viruses. Eur J Immunol 25:3256
44. Kalams SA, Johnson RP, Trocha AK, Dynan MJ, Ngo HS, DAquila RT, Kurnick JT, Walker BD (1994) Longitudinal analysis of T cell receptor (TCR) gene usage by human immunodeficiency virus 1 envelope-specific cytotoxic T lymphocyte clones reveals a limited TCR repertoire. J Exp Med 179:1261
45. Kannagi M, Chalifoux LV, Lord CI, Letvin NL (1988) Suppression of simian immunodeficiency virus replication in vitro by CD8[+] lymphocytes. J Immunol 140:2237
46. Kannagi M, Masuda T, Hattori T, Kanoh T, Nasu K, Yamamoto N, Harada S (1990) Interference with human immunodeficiency virus (HIV) replication by CD8[+] T cells in peripheral blood leukocytes of asymptomatic HIV carriers in vitro. J Immunol 65:3399
47. Kewalramani VN, Park CS, Gallombardo PA, Emerman M (1996) Protein stability influences human immunodeficiency virus type 2 Vpr virion incorporation and cell cycle effect. Virology 218:326
48. Klein MR, van Baalen C, Holwerda A, Kerkhof-Garde S, Bende R, Keet I, Eeftink-Schattenkerk J-K, Osterhaus A, Schuitemaker H, Miedema F (1995) Kinetics of Gag-specific cytotoxic T lymphocyte responses during the clinical course of HIV-1 infection: a longitudinal analysis of rapid progressors and long-term asymptomatics. J Exp Med 181:1356
49. Klenerman P, Rowland-Jones S, McAdam S, Edwards J, Daenke S, Lalloo D, Koppe B, Rosenberg W, Boyd D, Edwards A, Giangrande P, Phillips R, McMichael A (1994) Cytotoxic T cell activity antagonized by naturally occurring HIV-1 gag variants. Nature 369:403
50. Koup RA, Pikora CA, Luzuriaga K, Brettler DB, Day ES, Mazzara GP, Sullivan JL (1991) Limiting dilution analysis of cytotoxic T lymphocytes to human immunodeficiency virus gag antigens in infected persons: in vitro quantitation of effector cell pupulations with p17 and p24 specificities. J Exp Med 174:1593
51. Koup RA, Safrit JT, Cao Y, Andrews CA, McLeod G, Borkowsky W, Farthing C, Ho DD (1994) Temporal association of cellular immune responses with the initial control of viremia in primary human immunodeficiency virus type 1 syndrome. J Virol 68:4650
52. Lamhamedi-Cherradi S, Culmann-Penciolelli B, Guy B, Ly TD, Goujard C, Guillet JG, Gomard E (1995) Different patterns of HIV-1-specific cytotoxic T-lymphocyte activity after primary infection. AIDS 9:421
53. Levy J, Mackewicz C, Barker E (1996) Controlling HIV pathogenesis: the role of the noncytotoxic anti-HIV response of CD8[+] T cells. Immunol Today 17:217
54. Lowin B, Hahne M, Mattmann C, Tschopp J (1994) Cytolytic T-cell cytotoxicity is mediated through perforin and Fas lytic pathways. Nature 370:650
55. Mackewicz CE, Ortega HW, Levy JA (1991) CD8[+] cell anti-HIV activity correlates with the clinical state of the infected individual. J Clin Invest 87:1462
56. Mackewicz CE, Yang LC, Lifson JD, Levy JA (1994) Non-cytolytic CD8 T-cell anti-HIV responses in primary HIV-1 infection. Lancet 344:1671
57. Mackewicz CE, Blackbourn DJ, Levy JA (1995) CD8[+] T cells suppress human immunodeficiency virus replication by inhibiting viral transcription. Proc Natl Acad Sci USA 92:2308
58. Martz E, Howell D (1989) CTL: virus control first and cytolytic cells second? Immunol Today 10:79
59. Matloubian M, Conception RJ, Ahmed R (1994) CD4[+] T cells are required to sustain CD8[+] cytotoxic T-cell responses during chronic viral infection. J Virol 68:8056
60. McMichael AJ, Walker BD (1994) Cytotoxic T lymphocyte epitopes: implications for HIV vaccines. AIDS 8 [Suppl 1]:S155
61. McMichael AJ, Gotch FM, Cullen P, Askonas BA, Webster RG (1981) The human cytotoxic T cell response to influenza A vaccination. Clin Exp Immunol 43:276

62. Meier UC, Klenerman P, Griffin P, James W, Koppe B, Larder B, McMichael A, Phillips R (1995) Cytotoxic T lymphocyte lysis inhibited by viable HIV mutants. Science 270:1360
63. Mellors JW, Rinaldo CR Jr, Gupta P, White RM, Todd JA, Kingsley LA (1996) Prognosis in HIV-1 infection predicted by the quantity of virus in plasma. Science 272:1167
64. Meyerhans A, Dadaglio G, Vartanian J-P, Langlade-Demoyen P, Frank R, Asjö B, Plata F, Wain-Hobson S (1991) In vivo persistence of an HIV-1-encoded HLA-B27-restricted cytotoxic T lymphocyte epitope despite specific in vitro reactivity. Eur J Immunol 21:2637
65. Miedema F, Meyaard L, Koot M, et al (1994) Changing virus-host interactions in the course of HIV-1 infection. Immunol Rev 140:35
66. Moskophidis D, Zinkernagel RM (1995) Immunobiology of CTL escape mutants of LCMV. J Virol 69:2187
67. Moss PA, Rowland-Jones SL, Frodsham PM, McAdam S, Giangrande P, McMichael AJ, Bell JI (1995) Persistent high frequency of human immunodeficiency virus-specific cytotoxic T cells in peripheral blood of infected donors. Proc Natl Acad Sci USA 92:5773
68. Muller U, Steinhoff U, Reis LF, Hemmi S, Pavlovic J, Zinkernagel RM, Aguet M (1994) Functional role of type I and type II interferons in antiviral defense. Science 264:1918
69. Nietfield W, Bauer M, Fevrier M, Maier R, Holzwarth B, Frank R, Maier B, Riviere Y, Meyerhans A (1995) Sequence constraints and recognition by CTL of an HLA-B27-restricted HIV-1 gag epitope. J Immunol 154:2189
70. Nowak M, May RM, Phillips RE, Rowland-Jones S, Lalloo DG, McAdam S, Klenerman P, Koeppe B, Sigmund K, Bangham CRM, McMichael AJ (1995) Antigenic oscillations and shifting immunodominance in HIV-1 infections. Nature 375:606
71. O'Brien WA, Hartigan PM, Martin D, Esinhart J, Hill A, Benoit S, Rubin M, Simberkoff MS, Hailton JD (1996) Changes in plasma HIV-1 RNA and CD4$^+$ lymphocyte counts and the risk of progression to AIDS. Veterans Affairs Cooperative Study Group on AIDS. N Engl J Med 334:426
72. Pantaleo G, Graziosi C, Fauci AS (1993) New concepts in the immunopathogenesis of human immunodeficiency virus infection. N Engl J Med 328:327
73. Pantaleo G, Demarest JF, Soudeyns H, et al (1994) Major expansion of CD8$^+$ T cells with a predominant V beta usage during the primary immune response to HIV. Nature 370:463
74. Perelson AS, Neumann AU, Markowitz M, Leonard JM, Ho DD (1996) HIV-1 dynamics in vivo: virion clearance rate, infected cell life-span, and viral generation time. Science 271:1582
75. Pircher H, Moskophidis D, Rohrer U, Burki K, Hengartner H, Zinkernagel RM (1990) Viral escape by selection of cytotoxic T cell-resistant virus variants in vivo. Nature 346:629
76. Plata F, Autran B, Martins LP, Wain HS, Raphael M, Mayaud C, Denis M, Guillon JM, Debre P (1987) AIDS virus-specific cytotoxic T lymphocytes in lung disorders. Nature 328:348
77. Price P, Johnson RP, Scadden DT, Jassoy C, Rosenthal T, Kalams S, Walker BD (1995) Cytotoxic CD8$^+$ lymphocytes reactive with human immunodeficiency virus-1 produce granulocyte/macrophage colony-stimulating factor and variable amounts of interleukins 2, 3, and 4 following stimulation with the cognate epitope. Clin Immunol Immunopathol 74:100
78. Quinnan GVJ, Kirmani N, Rook AH, Manischewitz JF, Jackson L, Moreschi G, Santos GW Saral R, Burns WH (1982) Cytotoxic T cells in cytomegalovirus infection: HLA-restricted T-lymphocyte and non-T-lymphocyte cytotoxic responses correlate with recovery from cytomegalovirus infection in bone-marrow-transplant recipients. N Engl J Med 307:7
79. Racz P, Tenner-Racz K, Vloten F, Letvin N, Janossy G (1992) CD8$^+$ lymphocyte response in lymph nodes from patients with HIV infection. In: Racz P, Letvin N, Gluckman J (eds) Cytotoxic T cells in HIV and other retroviral infections. Karger, Basel, pp 162–173
80. Ramsay A, Ruby J, Ramshaw I (1993) A case for cytokines as effector molecules in the resolution of virus infection. Immunol Today 14:155
81. Reimann K, Tenner-Racz K, Racz P, Montefiori D, Yasutomi Y, Lin W, Ransil B, Letvin N (1994) Immunopathogenic events in acute infection of rhesus monkeys with simian immunodeficiency virus of macaques. J Virol 68:2362
82. Ringler D, Hancock W, King N, Letvin N, Daniel M, Derosiers R, Murphy G (1987) Immunophenotypic characterization of the cutaneous exanthem of SIV-infected rhesus monkeys. Am J Pathol 126:199
83. Riviere Y, Robertson MN, Buseyne F (1994) Cytotoxic T lymphocytes in human immunodeficiency virus infection: regulator genes (Review). Curr Top Microbiol Immunol 189:65

84. Saksela K, Stevens C, Rubinstein P, Baltimore D (1994) Human immunodeficiency virus type 1 mRNA expression in peripheral blood cells predicts disease progression independently of the numbers of CD4+ lymphocytes. Proc Natl Acad Sci USA 91:1104

85. Schwartz D, Sharma U, Busch M, Weinhold K, Matthews T, Lieberman J, Birx D, Farzedagen H, Margolick J, Quinn T, Davis B, Bagasra O, Pomerantz R, Viscidi R (1994) Absence of recoverable infectious virus and unique immune responses in an asymptomatic HIV+ long-term survivor. AIDS Res Hum Retroviruses 10:1703

85a. Sethi K, Naeher H, Stroehmann I (1988) Phenotypic heterogeneity of cerebrospinal fluid-derived HIV-specific and HLA-restricted cytotoxic T-cell clones. Nature 335:178–181

86. Sethi KK, Omata Y, Schneweis KE (1983) Protection of mice from fatal herpes simplex virus type 1 infection by adoptive transfer of cloned virus-specific and H-2-restricted cytotoxic T lymphocytes. J Gen Virol 64:443

86a. Takahashi K, Dai L, Fuerst T, Biddison W, Earl P, Moss B, Ennis F (1991) Specific lysis of human immunodeficiency virus type 1-infected cells by a HLA-A3.1-restricted CD8+ cytotoxic T-lymphocyte clone that recognizes a conserved peptide sequence within the gp41 subunit of the envelope protein. Proc Natl Acad Sci 88:10 277

87. Tenner-Racz K, Racz P, Thomé C, Meyer C, Anderson P, Schlossman S, Letvin N (1993) Cytotoxic effector cell granules recognized by the monoclonal antibody TIA-1 are present in CD8+ lymphocytes in lymph nodes of human immunodeficiency virus-1-infected patients. Am J Pathol 142:1750

88. Tsubota H, Lord CI, Watkins DI, Morimoto C, Letvin NL (1989) A cytotoxic T lymphocyte inhibits acquired immunodeficiency syndrome virus replication in peripheral blood lymphocytes. J Exp Med 169:1421

89. Von Herrath M, Oldstone MB, Fox HS (1995) Simian immunodeficiency virus (SIV)-specific CTL in cerebrospinal fluid and brains of SIV-infected rhesus macaques. J Immunol 154:5582

90. Von Herrath MG, Yokoyama M, Dockter J, Oldstone MB, Whitton JL (1996) CD4-deficient mice have reduced levels of memory cytotoxic T lymphocytes after immunization and show diminished resistance to subsequent virus challenge. J Virol 70:1072

91. Walker BD, Chakrabarti S, Moss B, Paradis TJ, Flynn T, Durno AG, Blumberg RS, Kaplan JC, Hirsch MS, Schooley RT (1987) HIV-specific cytotoxic T lymphocytes in seropositive individuals. Nature 328:345

92. Walker CM, Moody DJ, Stites DP, Levy JA (1986) CD8+ lymphocytes can control HIV infection in vitro by suppressing virus replication. Science 234:1563

93. Walker CM, Erickson AL, Hsueh FC, Levy JA (1991) Inhibition of human immunodeficiency virus replication in acutely infected CD4+ cells by CD8+ cells involves a noncytotoxic mechanism. J Virol 65:5921

94. Walker CM, Thomson HGA, Hsueh FC, Erickson AL, Pan LZ, Levy JA (1991) CD8+ T cells from HIV-1-infected individuals inhibit acute infection by human and primate immunodeficiency viruses. Cell Immunol 137:420

95. Walter E, Greenberg P, Gilbert M, Finch R, Watanabe K, Thomas E, Riddell S (1995) Reconstitution of cellular immunity against cytomegalovirus in recipients of allogeneic bone marrow by transfer of T-cell clones from the donor. N Engl Med 333:1038

96. Yamamoto H, Ringler DJ, Miller MD, Yasutomi Y, Hasunuma T, Letvin NL (1992) Simian immunodeficiency virus-specific cytotoxic T lymphocytes are present in the AIDS-associated skin rash in rhesus monkeys. J Immunol 149:728

97. Yang OO, Johnson RP, Kalams SA, Trocha A, Walker BD (1996) HIV-1-specific cytotoxic T lymphocytes inhibit HIV-1 replication by specific and non-specific mechanisms. In: Abstracts of the XI International AIDS Conference. Vancouver, 1996

98. Yang OO, Kalams SA, Rosenzweig M, Trocha A, Jones N, Koziel M, Walker BD, Johnson RP (1996) Efficient lysis of HIV-1 infected cells by cytotoxic T lymphocytes. J Virol 70:5799

99. Yap KL, Ada GL, McKenzie IF (1978) Transfer of specific cytotoxic T lymphocytes protects mice inoculated with influenza virus. Nature 273:238

100. York IA, Roop C, Andrews DW, Riddell SR, Graham FL, Johnson DC (1994) A cytosolic herpes simplex virus protein inhibits antigen presentation to CD8+ T lymphocytes. Cell 77:525

101. Zinkernagel RM, Althage A (1977) Antiviral protection by virus-immune cytotoxic T cells. Infected target cells are lysed before infectious virus progeny is assembled. J Exp Med 145:644

102. Zinkernagel RM, Hengartner H (1994) T-cell-mediated immunopathology versus direct cytolysis by virus: implications for HIV and AIDS (Review). Immunol Today 15:262

Noncytolytic CD8 T cell-mediated suppression of HIV replication

Michael L. Greenberg, Simon F. Lacey, Chin-Ho Chen, Dani P. Bolognesi, Kent J. Weinhold

Department of Surgery, Box 2926, Duke University Medical Center, Durham, NC 27710, USA

Introduction

Infection with the human immunodeficiency virus type 1 (HIV-1) usually results in a progressive immunodeficiency disease culminating in the development of AIDS [4, 28, 39]. A small subset of infected individuals has been described who do not exhibit immunosuppression or disease for prolonged periods [10, 38, 56]. Although attenuated strains of HIV-1 are associated with some cohorts of long-term non-progressors [34, 46], strong immune responses and low virus loads noted with other cohorts [11, 49] raise the possibility that specific and/or particularly effective antiviral immune responses may confer long-lasting protection. This chapter focuses on a cellular immune response that may comprise one element of a protective response to HIV-1 infection, CD8$^+$ T cell-mediated noncytolytic suppression of HIV.

Primary infection with HIV-1 is frequently associated with an acute clinical viral syndrome [57], and characterized by extensive virus replication and dissemination, resulting in high levels of plasma viremia [1, 14, 19]. Within a short period of time (days to a few weeks), infected individuals mount vigorous humoral and cellular antiviral immune responses evidenced by seroconversion to HIV-1 antigens, generation of antibodies that mediate cellular cytotoxicity, and the presence of HIV-1-specific cytotoxic T lymphocytes (CTL) in the peripheral blood compartment [23, 36]. Development of these immune responses is accompanied by dramatic decreases in plasma viremia and resolution of the acute clinical syndrome. The ensuing asymptomatic phase of HIV-1 disease generally lasts for years, with a mean time from infection to progression to AIDS estimated at 10 years [48]. The vigorous humoral and cellular immune responses of HIV-1-infected individuals are thought to contribute substantially to curtailing the acute viremic phase and establishing and maintaining the asymptomatic state.

Virus replication occurs throughout the prolonged asymptomatic phase with large numbers of virus-infected cells residing in lymphoid tissues [24, 47, 50, 52]. The

---

Correspondence to: M.L. Greenberg

course of HIV-1 disease is determined largely by the level of virus expression as evidenced by studies examining various markers of viral load [11, 17, 24, 26, 30, 45, 47, 49, 50, 52, 55], including the studies of Mellors et al. [44] and Hogervorst et al. [31], in which the levels of plasma viral RNA, measured approximately 1 year after primary infection, were found to be predictive for clinical progression over the ensuing 5 years. Although it has not been possible to demonstrate which elements of the immune response to HIV-1 infection constitute "protective immunity", the central role of virus replication in disease progression argues that protective responses will limit HIV-1 expression in vivo. Neutralizing antibody responses generally develop after plasma viremia has already diminished [23, 36]. Although antibodies that mediate antibody-dependent cellular cytotoxicity (ADCC) do develop particularly early in primary infection [23], their role in limiting HIV-1 activity in vivo remains to be established. Thus far, it appears that cellular immune responses, particularly major histocompatibility complex (MHC) class I-restricted HIV-1-specific CTL, are most closely associated with decreased virus expression in vivo.

Observations suggesting that cellular immune responses may limit virus replica-. tion and spread in infected individuals include the considerable body of work demonstrating that CTL displaying specificities for many viral-encoded products are readily detected during the asymptomatic phase of disease (reviewed in [60]). A role for virus-specific CTL responses in the control of virus expression has also been inferred from studies demonstrating that these responses wane as infected individuals progress to AIDS. Furthermore, Koup et al. [36] and Borrow et al. [6], both found a temporal relationship between the appearance of anti-HIV-1 CTL and resolution of plasma viremia during the acute phase of infection, as well as an inverse relationship between detectable CTL reactivity and plasma viremia.

In addition to their MHC class I-restricted antigen-specific anti-HIV-1 CTL effector function, an important and often ignored activity of CD8 cells, noncytolytic suppression of HIV-1, was originally described a decade ago by Walker et al. [62]. Until quite recently, the nature of this inhibitory activity and its role as a component of protective immunity remained controversial. It is now apparent from the results of many laboratories that CD8 cells from asymptomatic infected individuals can potently inhibit HIV-1 replication through noncytolytic mechanisms. Moreover, within the past year, important findings identified β-chemokines as soluble mediators of virus-suppressive activity [15], and that fusin [27] and the β-chemokine receptor C-C CKR-5 [21, 22] were accessory molecules required for virus-cell fusion, providing fresh insights into mechanisms of noncytolytic inhibition. The coalescence of the previously distinct fields of noncytolytic CD8 virus suppression, proinflamatory chemotactic cytokines (i.e., chemokines), virus fusion, and G-protein-coupled receptors has fostered explosive growth in efforts to understand their relationships to HIV-1 infection. In this article, we review and update our current understanding of CD8 virus-suppressive activity, and indicate aspects of this antiviral activity which remain to be elucidated. We also outline areas needing definition if this immune reactivity is to be employed in preventive and/or interventive strategies.

CD8⁺ T lymphocyte-mediated inhibition of HIV-1 replication

The ability of CD8⁺ cells to suppress HIV-1 replication through noncytolytic mechanisms became apparent from studies of Walker et al. [62] and later of other investigators [7], which demonstrated that virus recovery from activated peripheral blood mononuclear cells (PBMC) of infected individuals sometimes required, and was often augmented by, the specific depletion of CD8⁺ lymphocytes prior to activation. Walker et al. [63] further demonstrated that addition of the removed CD8⁺ lymphocytes to the CD8⁺-depleted cultures resulted in a dose-dependent inhibition of HIV-1 replication, verifying the virus-suppressive activity of CD8⁺ cells. In addition to its presence in HIV-1-infected humans, CD8⁺ noncytolytic inhibition of immunodeficiency virus replication is prevalent in animal model systems [33]. Particularly potent CD8⁺ inhibitory activity has been noted in the simian immunodeficiency virus (SIV)smm-infected sooty mangabey system [54], the SIVagm-infected African green monkey model [25], and the HIV-1-infected chimpanzee [12]. Interestingly, infection in these animal models does not result in manifestation of disease.

Assay systems to examine CD8⁺ suppression of HIV-1

The ability of CD8⁺ T cell effectors to suppress HIV-1 replication is usually studied in systems employing mitogen- or antibody-activated primary CD4⁺ lymphocytes targets. Virus replication is either initiated by activation of proviral genomes with naturally infected cells in endogenous assays, which employ CD4⁺ targets obtained from infected individuals, or de novo by in vitro infection of CD4⁺ targets from seronegative donors with cell-free virus in acute assays [7, 62, 64]. Autologous or heterologous activated CD8⁺ effectors can be examined with either assay system. The endogenous assay is useful for detecting inhibitory activity with autologous infected cells, but limited for purposes of quantifying suppressive activity, especially with samples from different individuals, due to the inability to standardize virus challenge as well as target cells. Nevertheless, studies employing the endogenous assay have found CD8⁺-suppressive activity correlating with the clinical disease stage, prompting suggestions that the activity may be important for sustaining the asymptomatic state [29, 40].

The acute assay allows the standardization of virus inocula and target cells and is better suited for quantitative assessments. It also permits examination of suppressive activity with HIV-1 strains of differing phenotypes and/or genotypes. In the acute assays, only CD8⁺ cells obtained from HIV-1-infected individuals inhibit virus replication, in contrast to endogenous assays where CD8⁺ effectors from uninfected as well as infected individuals can suppress [8, 40, 63, 64]. The distinct results with the endogenous versus acute system may suggest that various CD8⁺ inhibitory mechanisms operate. In addition, the results may reflect differing sensitivities to CD8⁺-suppressive reactivities for the challenge viruses employed in the two systems (see below). Recently, Barker et al. [3] described CD8⁺-suppressive activity with a model system designed to mimic the microenvironment within lymphoid organs based upon interactions between dendritic cells and non-activated CD4⁺ cells. Two sets of CD8⁺-suppressive activities were identified with variations of the system employing natural and in vitro infected CD4⁺ target cells. With endogenous assays, they found that suppressive activity reflected immune competence, as potent inhibitory activity was detected with CD8$^+$ effectors from seronegative and early-stage-infected subjects but not with effectors from late-stage AIDS subjects. In acute assays with the dendritic cell-CD4$^+$ cell system, CD8$^+$ virus-inhibitory activity reflected a response to HIV-1-infection, with potent suppression occurring with effectors from infected subjects regardless of disease stage, whereas inhibitory activity was not observed with cells from seronegative subjects [3].

Suppression of HIV-1 replication by noncytolytic mechanisms

Initial studies of CD8$^+$ virus-suppressive activity suggested that inhibition was not a result of CTL effector function. CD8$^+$-mediated inhibition of HIV-1 replication did not involve elimination of HIV-1-infected cells, nor was it accompanied by cytolysis of HIV-1-infected CD4$^+$ targets [64]. In addition, the inhibitory activity was observed with heterologous effectors and targets, suggesting that it was not restricted by MHC class I antigens [8, 64]. However, this issue remained controversial as studies with SIV-infected rhesus macaques suggested that CD8$^+$ suppression was restricted by MHC class I antigens and mediated by a CTL [59]. We have examined this issue from several perspectives with results that lead us to conclude that CTL reactivities and suppression of HIV-1 are indeed separable. In one set of studies we found that proviral DNA copy number does not decrease when virus replication and viral RNA levels are suppressed by CD8$^+$ cells, implying a non-lytic mechanism [13]. In other studies designed to characterize the effector cells mediating CD8$^+$-suppression, panels of CD8$^+$ cell clones were derived from HIV-1-infected individuals, and examined for CTL reactivity against *env*, *gag*, *pol* and *nef*-targeted B lymphocyte cell lines (BLCL), in addition to virus-suppressive activity. The clonal nature of the cells was confirmed by analysis of T cell receptor (TCR) Vβ gene expression. CD8$^+$ clones were recovered that exhibited virus-suppression but were devoid of detectable HIV-1-specific CTL reactivity, in addition to clones devoid of suppressive activity with demonstrable HIV-1-specific CTL [58]. CD8$^+$ clones were also recovered that either exhibited or lacked both activities. Thus, CD8$^+$-suppression and HIV-specific CTL activities in some cases were separated at the clonal level, although the activities were not mutually exclusive [58]. Virus-suppressive CD8$^+$ clones were heterogeneous with respect to phenotypic markers and TCR Vβ gene expression, indicating that suppressive reactivities are oligoclonal. Similar suppressive reactivities in CD8$^+$ cell clones have also been reported by Hsueh et al. [32].

    In another approach, we generated a stable transformed CD8$^+$ cell line from primary bulk suppressive cells [37] with the 488–77 strain of Herpesvirus saimiri (HVS) [5]. CTL assays employing Epstein-Barr virus-transformed BLCL infected with vaccinia constructs expressing the HIV-1 *env*, *gag*, *pol* and *nef* proteins as targets were unable to detect significant HLA-restricted cytolysis with this cell line despite using a high ratio of effector to target cells. Comparison of the virus inhibitory activity of the HVS-transformed CD8$^+$ cells with primary non-transformed CD8$^+$ cells from the same patient demonstrated that the transformed CD8$^+$ cells were very similar to the primary CD8$^+$ cells in their ability to inhibit HIV-1 production from autologous CD4$^+$ cells [37]. Moreover, when tested against infected CD4$^+$ targets from an HIV-1$^+$ patient completely mismatched for MHC class I alleles, potent inhibition was observed indicating, together with the lack of detectable CTL reactivity, that virus inhibition by the transformed CD8$^+$ cell line was not due to MHC class I-restricted CTL activity.

Noncytolytic inhibition of HIV-1 mediated by soluble factors

The lack of definitive information regarding the nature of the effector mechanism(s) by which CD8+ cells inhibit HIV-1 replication has, until recently, hampered appreciation of its role in HIV-1-infection. At least part of the effector mechanism appears to be due to secretion of soluble factors from CD8+ cells. The soluble inhibitory activity was originally demonstrated in studies in which CD8+ cells suppressed virus production even when physically separated from infected CD4+ target cells by a semipermeable membrane [61]. Other studies confirmed the presence of a soluble mediator by demonstrating HIV-1 inhibitory activity in medium conditioned by CD8+ cells [8]. Inhibition of virus replication by CD8+ cell-derived soluble components has also been observed with the dendritic cell-CD4+ cell system [3]. However, the highly potent CD8+ cell-mediated inhibition of HIV-1 has not been fully reproduced with CD8+ cell-derived soluble materials in either the PBMC-based or the dendritic cell system. The issue of whether CD8+ cell-associated virus-suppressive activity is solely mediated by soluble factors, or if additional mechanisms requiring contact of the CD8+ effector cell with the CD4+ target are operative remains unresolved, but in need of clarification. Further considerations regarding this issue are described below.

Efforts to identify the soluble inhibitory components have been ongoing since the late 1980s. A number of cytokines exhibiting complex interactions are known to modulate HIV-1 expression in various systems [53]. Studies by Mackewicz et al. [41] and Brinchmann et al. [9] had, however, suggested that the active CD8+-derived components were distinct from known cytokines. Progress towards uncovering the nature of the soluble factor(s) was hindered by the absence of systems capable of generating sufficient quantities of material for purification purposes, and also by deficiencies in the assays employed. Cocchi et al. [15] addressed these problems by examining HTLV-1-transformed CD8+ cell clones with a highly sensitive assay that they developed. Using these systems, Gallo's group identified the chemotactic cytokines RANTES, MIP-1α and MIP-1β as the major HIV-1 inhibitors in CD8+ cell culture supernatants [15]. Employing an HIV-1 suppression assay based on the HUT78 T cell line-derived PM-1 cells, they demonstrated HIV-1-inhibitory activity with β-chemokines purified from the culture supernatants of an HTLV-1-transformed CD8+ cell clone. In the PM-1 system, nanogram concentrations per milliliter of recombinant RANTES, MIP-1α or MIP-1β were shown to inhibit HIV-1 replication. In addition, they found that neutralizing antibodies to all three chemokines used together effectively abrogated the inhibitory activity of culture supernatants from the HTLV-1-transformed CD8+ cell clone and activated primary CD8+ cells from HIV-1+ asymptomatic individuals. In contrast, when the antibodies were used individually, inhibitory activity was not blocked, prompting their conclusion that the three β-chemokines were the major HIV-suppressive factors from CD8+ cells [15].

The identification of HIV-suppressive factors released from CD8+ cells opened new directions for investigating the biology of CD8+ cell antiviral activities. However, the finding that greater than 100-fold higher concentrations of the recombinant β-chemokines were required to effect virus inhibition with primary CD4+ targets, as compared with PM-1 cells [15], also raised questions concerning the role of the β-chemokines as mediators of CD8+ virus-suppressive activity in primary CD4+ T lymphocytes. Moreover, while activated primary CD8+ cells from HIV-1+ asymptomatic individuals produced seemingly sufficient levels of the β-chemokines to account for

HIV-1 inhibition in the PM-1 system, the observed levels appeared insufficient to account for inhibitory activity with primary cell targets [15].

Working with primary CD4$^+$ T lymphocytes, Baier et al. [2] reported HIV-1-inhibitory activity associated with another chemotactic cytokine produced by CD8$^+$ cells, IL-16. Relatively high concentrations of recombinant human IL-16 were necessary to inhibit virus production from primary cells. These investigators had also cloned and examined the activity of IL-16 from African green monkey cells. Although the sequence of human IL-16 was very similar to the African green monkey homolog, it was three to four orders of magnitude less potent in inhibiting HIV-1 replication [2]. Currently, the relationship between IL-16 and the soluble CD8$^+$ factor that suppresses activity is unclear.

Prior to the reports from Gallo's group [15] and Kurth's laboratory [2], we had found that soluble factors secreted from the HVS-transformed CD8$^+$ cell line described above inhibit HIV-1 production in primary CD4$^+$ cells [37]. We concentrated the suppressive activity from large volumes of serum-free conditioned medium by more than 200-fold, and subjected the material to size fractionation using fast protein liquid chromatography with a Superdex 200 column. The fractions were examined for suppressive activity and cytotoxicity using assays employing primary CD4$^+$ cells and virus isolates, and analyzed by sodium dodecyl sulfate-polyacrylamide gel electrophoresis under reducing conditions. We noted that peak virus-suppressive activity was recovered in fractions exhibiting one major silver-stained band migrating at a relative molecular weight of approximately 8000. Neither overt toxicity nor growth inhibitory effects were observed with the HVS-transformed cell-derived conditioned medium or active fractions derived from concentrates (S.F.L. and M.L.G., in preparation).

The report by Cocchi et al. [15] identifying the β-chemokines as the major HIV-1-suppressive factors from CD8$^+$ cells [15], and the similarities between the molecular weights for RANTES, MIP-1α, and MIP-1β (approximately 7800, 7600, and 7800, respectively) with that estimated for the major band associated with the fractions showing peak activity from the Superdex 200 column, led us to investigate whether these β-chemokines were components of the active fractions. Western blot analysis with monospecific polyclonal goat antibodies demonstrated that RANTES, MIP-1α and MIP-1β were indeed present in the active fractions. Further separation of pooled active fractions by reverse phase chromatography as described in [15], demonstrated that RANTES, MIP-1α and MIP-1β [determined by Western blotting and enzyme-linked immunosorbent assay (ELISA)] remained associated with virus-suppressive fractions (S.F.L. and M.L.G., in preparation).

To examine whether these compounds were responsible for CD8$^+$-suppressive activity with primary CD4$^+$ cells, we performed antibody blocking experiments with polyclonal neutralizing antibodies against each of the three chemokines to discern if they would abrogate the virus inhibitory effect of the unfractionated soluble concentrate described above, as well as the activity of the HVS-transformed CD8$^+$ cells. For these experiments, we used an amount of the soluble concentrate sufficient to cause a 1 log reduction in infectivity, or a 1:1 ratio of CD8$^+$ effector cells to CD4$^+$ targets. Anti-chemokine antibodies were tested either individually or together to attempt abrogation of virus-inhibitory activity. In addition, we examined monoclonal anti-chemokine antibodies in some assays to employ higher chemokine neutralizing titers. Representative results from these experiments are depicted in Fig. 1. The soluble concentrate completely inhibited infection with an inocula of 200 median tissue culture

Effect of Anti-chemokine Antibodies on CD8 Suppression and Virus Replication

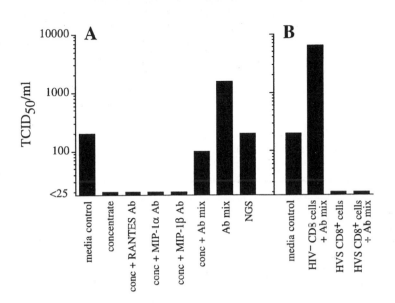

Fig. 1A, B. β-Chemokine neutralizing antibodies block suppressive activity of CD8$^+$ cell-derived soluble materials but not activity of CD8$^+$ cells. Primary CD4$^+$ cells were purified from blood samples from normal donors and activated with phytohemagglutinin for 3 days prior to infection with the QZ4734 primary isolate. **A** Concentrated supernatants (*concentrate* or *conc*) from a Herpesvirus saimiri (HVS)-transformed CD8$^+$ cell line were added to the cultures at a final concentration of 10% (v/v) at the time of infection, where indicated. Chemokine neutralizing antibodies (*Ab*), included as indicated, were incubated with concentrated supernatants for 1 h prior to addition; 300 μg/ml anti-RANTES, and 100 μg/ml of anti-MIP-1α and MIP-1β polyclonal neutralizing antibodies were present during the preincubation. *Ab mix* indicates the combined use of antibodies to RANTES, MIP-1α and MIP-1β. Virus replication was monitored by assaying for release of reverse transcriptase activity [13]. **B** CD8$^+$ cells purified from normal donors or the HVS-transformed CD8$^+$ cells were added where indicated at a final ratio of 1:1 with respect to the CD4$^+$ targets, at the time of infection. β-Chemokine neutralizing antibodies were used at the concentrations indicated for **A**, and preincubations of antibodies with CD8$^+$ effectors took place for 1 h prior to addition to cultures

infective dose (TCID$_{50}$) of a primary isolate (Fig. 1A). Although the anti-chemokine antibodies used individually were without effect on the activity of the concentrate, a mixture of all three anti-chemokine neutralizing antibodies caused infectivity to return almost to the levels observed in the absence of added CD8$^+$ concentrate or chemokine antibodies (Fig. 1A, 6th column from the left), reproducing the results reported by Cocchi et al. [15] that led to their conclusion that these β-chemokines were the major HIV-1-suppressive factors from CD8$^+$ cells.

Although the work from Gallo's group has focused attention on β-chemokine production from CD8$^+$ cells, RANTES was originally considered to be the product of mature CD4$^+$ cells, and CD4$^+$ cells produce significant levels of MIP-1α, and MIP-1β, in addition to RANTES [16]. When we examined the effects on virus infectivity of only the mixture of anti-β-chemokine antibodies, we observed a 16-fold increase in virus titer (Fig. 1A, 7th column from the left), suggesting that production of the β-chemokines by activated primary CD4$^+$ cells may be sufficient to influence HIV-1-

infection. Similar implications are evident in the experiment depicted in Fig. 1B (2nd column from left), where the combination of anti-chemokine antibodies resulted in a 64-fold increase in the observed virus titer. We have found that increased virus infection of CD4$^+$ cells with anti-β-chemokine antibodies is dependent on the particular target cells examined. CD4$^+$ cells from some donors exhibit marked increases in virus titer when treated with all three chemokine neutralizing antibodies, whereas the effects are much more modest, and in some cases not detectable, with other preparations of CD4$^+$ cells. Recently, Paxton et al. [51] have found that CD4$^+$ cells from two HIV-1-exposed uninfected individuals resist infection with certain strains of HIV-1. They demonstrated that the cells secreted highly elevated levels of RANTES, and lesser amounts of MIP-1α and MIP-1β, causing speculation that β-chemokine production by CD4$^+$ cells may influence the outcome of encounters with HIV-1. Although it is not clear whether β-chemokine production by the CD4$^+$ cells from the exposed uninfected individuals is directly responsible for their resistance to HIV-1-infection [22], these investigators have demonstrated that release of β-chemokines from these CD4$^+$ cells is sufficient to inhibit HIV-1 replication in bystander CD4$^+$ cells [22].

The implication of these results are significant, not only for HIV-1 biology, but they perhaps confound interpretation of the antibody-blocking experiments described above with the soluble concentrate and primary CD4$^+$ cells. Comparison of viral titer in the presence of the chemokine antibody mixture alone in Fig. 1A (3200 TCID$_{50}$) with that observed when the soluble concentrate is added with the mixture of antibodies (100 TCID$_{50}$) may indicate that other components contribute to virus inhibition. Moreover, as shown in Fig. 1B, we found that the anti-chemokine antibodies were unable to exert any blocking effect on the inhibitory activity of the CD8$^+$ cells (compare 3rd and 4th columns from left), although quantification of β-chemokine levels by ELISA suggested the antibodies were present in excess. These results indicate that the β-chemokines may not be the sole mediators of CD8$^+$ noncytolytic suppressive activity. A similar conclusion was reached by Barker et al. [3] with the dendritic cell-CD4$^+$ cell system, in which CD8$^+$-suppressive activity could not be fully accounted for by the β-chemokines. Collectively these studies have confirmed the antiviral activity associated with RANTES, MIP-1α and MIP-1β described by Gallo's group, but also suggested that other components may be significant contributors to CD8$^+$ virus-suppression in primary CD4$^+$ cells.

Table 1. Inhibitory activity of CD8-derived concentrate against laboratory and primary HIV-1 isolates Percentage (v/v) of CD8-derived concentrate required to reduce infectious titer

Virus	$V_n/V_0 = 0.1$	$V_n/V_0 = 0.02$
QZ4734	< 1%	1.7%
NL4-3	> 25%	> 25%

Virus stocks of the QZ4734 primary isolate and NL4-3 molecular clone were titered on activated primary CD4$^+$ cells in the presence or absence of serial dilutions of a concentrated supernatant from a Herpesvirus saimiri-transformed CD8$^+$ cell line. Virus replication was monitored by assaying for release of reverse transcriptase [13], and the concentration of supernatant required to inhibit infectivity by the amounts indicated were determined by interpolation

Distinct susceptibility to β-chemokine-mediated inhibition among HIV-1 isolates is determined by accessory molecules required for virus fusion

An important finding in the report by Cocchi et al. [15] demonstrated the insensitivity of the IIIB/LAI laboratory strain of HIV to inhibition by RANTES, MIP-1α, and MIP-1β. We have examined this issue with a quantitative infectivity reduction assay, adapted from antibody neutralization studies, to compare the inhibition of several HIV-1 isolates by the HVS-transformed CD8$^+$ cell-derived concentrate. A common set of CD4$^+$ targets were employed in two-dimensional assays with infectious virus titered in one dimension, and the concentrated CD8$^+$ supernatant in the other dimension. We determined the supernatant concentration required to reduce virus infectivity by either 10-fold ($V_n/V_0 = 0.1$) or 50-fold ($V_n/V_0 = 0.02$) (Table 1). Infectivity of the primary isolate QZ4734, was reduced by 50-fold with approximately 2% final concentration of the β-chemokine-containing concentrate (Table 1). The QZ4734 primary isolate employed is a low-passage (P1) isolate recovered from an individual early during acute infection, and behaves similarly in these assays to several other low-passage primary isolates. In contrast, neither the infectivity nor level of viral replication of the NL4-3 molecular clone was significantly affected even with a 25% final concentration of the β-chemokine containing material. In addition, we reproduced the findings of Cocchi et al. [15] with the IIIB/LAI isolate, and found that the prototypic HIV-1 RF isolate is also insensitive to β-chemokine-mediated inhibition. In general, we have found that laboratory strains are resistant to inhibition by β-chemokines, whereas most, although not all, low-passage primary isolates are sensitive. The resistance of the prototypic isolates could not be ascribed to differences in virus replication kinetics, nor to the source cells used to prepare the virus stocks. Using the quantitative suppression assay described above, we have also found differing sensitivities among primary isolates. The resistance of the NL4-3 molecular clone to inhibition by RANTES, MIP-1α, and MIP-1β has recently been reported by Dragic et al. [22] and by Deng et al. [21]. These data provide convincing evidence for the existence of viral determinants of sensitivity to β-chemokine inhibition.

Explanations for these findings have been provided by a series of recent reports originating from an unexpected area of HIV-1 biology, HIV-1 envelope-mediated virus fusion. Although the CD4$^+$ molecule was demonstrated as the principal receptor for HIV-1 [20, 35], it has been known for some time that CD4$^+$ by itself was not sufficient for infection to occur, and it was suspected that another molecule or "second receptor" might be involved [43]. Despite many years spent by a number of laboratories searching for the elusive "second receptor", clarification of its nature was not forthcoming until an elegant and important series of experiments were reported by Feng et al. [27]. Pursuing studies of virus fusion for a number of years, these investigators adapted a transient expression fusion assay employing recombinant vaccinia virus vectors that they had developed to screen a cDNA library for a fusion cofactor permitting a CD4$^+$-expressing non-human cell to undergo HIV-1 envelope-mediated fusion. Using this system for functional expression cloning, they identified a gene for a molecule they term "fusin", based on its ability to serve as a fusion cofactor, and demonstrated its role in the process of HIV-1 envelope-mediated viral fusion [27]. Sequence analysis indicated that the gene belonged to a family of G-protein-coupled receptors, and that its sequence encoded an "orphan-receptor" most similar to the receptor for the α-chemokine IL-8 [27]. Furthermore, Berger's group demonstrated that fusin preferentially enabled laboratory strains of HIV-1, in contrast to primary or macrophage-tropic strains, to infect cells [27]. Thus, fusin, an α-chemokine receptor is required for infection by the same types of HIV-1 isolates that were insensitive to inhibition by the β-chemokines. Berger's group speculated on the probability that other molecules required for fusion of macrophage-tropic isolates existed, and hypothesized that a receptor for RANTES, MIP-1α and MIP-1β might serve as a fusion cofactor for macrophage-tropic isolates. Building on the findings from Berger's group, and the work from Gallo's laboratory, collaborative efforts between investigators at the Aaron Diamond AIDS Research Center, Progenics Pharmaceuticals, DNAX Research Institute, Stanford University Medical Center, University of Louisville School of Medicine, and the Skirball and Howard Hughes Institutes at NYU Medical Center have demonstrated that a β-chemokine receptor that binds RANTES, MIP-1α, and MIP-1β, termed C-C CKR-5, permits fusion and entry of macrophage-tropic isolates [22, 23], verifying the hypothesis put forth by Berger's group. These studies also indicate that the β-chemokines inhibit HIV-1 infection by blocking the post-CD4 binding fusion process [21, 22]. Thus, the antiviral activity of the β-chemokines described by Cocchi et al. [15] is due to effects on virus entry mediated by the receptor for the β-chemokines. The results help to explain the selectivity of the β-chemokines for primary or macrophage-tropic isolates versus prototypic or cell line adapted isolates. The studies of Deng et al. [21] and Dragic et al. [22] also demonstrate that sensitivity to the β-chemokines, and use of C-C CKR-5 for virus entry, is determined by the ectodomain of the viral envelope glycoprotein. Although the precise sequences involved have not been identified, the association of susceptibility to the β-chemokines with viral tropism implicates the V3 region as one possible determinant for sensitivity to β-chemokine inhibition. A model depicting virus entry of prototypic (designated SI for syncytia-inducing) and primary (designated NSI for non-syncytia-inducing) strains of HIV-1, and selective inhibition by the β-chemokines is presented in Fig. 2. A possibility suggested by the results described above, and implied in Fig. 2, is that the natural ligand for fusin may exhibit selective inhibitory activity for prototypic/SI variants of HIV.

Other mechanisms for suppression of HIV-1 by CD8$^+$ cells

We have indicated above that there are quantitative as well as qualitative differences in virus-suppression mediated by CD8$^+$ cells versus their derived soluble materials. A number of studies have indicated that CD8$^+$ cells inhibit replication of prototypic strains of HIV-1, albeit perhaps not as efficiently as primary isolates, and we have illustrated above that CD8$^+$ cells inhibit primary isolates even in the presence of chemokine-neutralizing antibodies. These observations, as well as the distinct suppressive reactivities found with endogenous and acute suppression assays [3, 8, 40, 63, 64], suggest that several noncytolytic inhibitory mechanisms may be used by CD8$^+$ cells to control HIV-1 replication.

The specific decreases in viral RNA occurring during CD8$^+$ cell-mediated suppression suggested to us the possibility that CD8$^+$ effectors may directly influence virus gene expression [13]. It appears that down-regulation of transcriptional activity from the HIV-1 long terminal repeat (LTR) promoter may be involved in the HIV-1-inhibitory activity associated with CD8$^+$ cells. Studies from our group first demonstrated that CD8$^+$ cells from asymptomatic HIV-1-infected individuals inhibited the activity of the HIV-1 LTR in a natural host cell for the virus, the primary CD4$^+$ T lymphocyte [13]. Inhibition of HIV-1 LTR-driven transcription occurred in either

SI

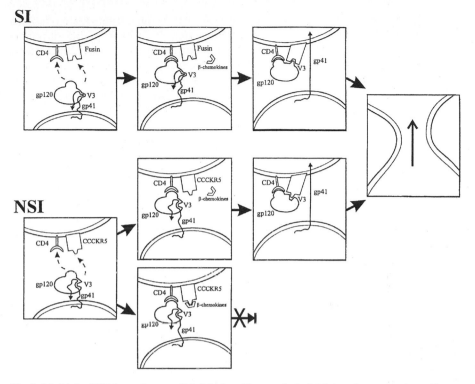

NSI

Fig. 2. Model for HIV-1 envelope-mediated fusion. *Top panels* depict interactions occurring with envelope glycoproteins of syncytia-inducing (*SI*) isolates and cellular components, and *bottom panels* depict analogous interactions between virus envelope glycoproteins of non-syncytia-inducing (*NSI*) isolates and cellular components. Schema based on [15, 22, 23, 27]

the presence or absence of the transcriptional transactivator *tat*, and was not subject to MHC class I restriction [13]. Transcriptional inhibitory activity for the HIV-1 LTR was limited to CD8+ effectors from HIV-infected individuals, and was also demonstrated with medium conditioned by CD8+ cells [13]. These findings have largely been confirmed in studies from Mackewicz et al. [42] and Copeland et al. [18]. Whether the observed inhibition of HIV LTR promoter activity by CD8+ effectors comprises a significant mechanism by which CD8+ cells suppress virus replication remains to be determined.

Conclusions

Significant advances have occurred in our understanding of noncytolytic CD8+ cell-mediated virus suppression. The β-chemokines RANTES, MIP-1α, and MIP-1β have been identified as soluble mediators of virus suppression, and their mechanism of action is being elucidated. Importantly, the discovery of accessory molecules required for virus fusion [21, 22, 27] has profoundly impacted the way we view noncytolytic suppressive activities, and suggests new therapeutic and preventive strategies for HIV-1 disease. However, considerable work remains for future studies to provide the insights necessary to take advantage of noncytolytic inhibitory reactivities. Currently, knowledge concerning induction of virus-suppressive activity is quite limited, although this information will be critical for preventive strategies. In this regard, studies of noncytolytic activities in individuals experiencing primary infection as well as volunteers receiving vaccine candidates should prove illuminating. Few studies have investigated whether infection with other viral agents leads to similar noncytolytic activities.

In connection with possible therapeutic strategies, it will be important to determine whether relationships exist between the switch from NSI to SI variants, which often accompanies disease progression, and the endogenous activity of the β-chemokines. Further definition of the full spectrum of noncytolytic inhibitory mechanisms and molecules of CD8$^+$ cells, and their soluble factors, will also be helpful. The finding that accessory molecules required for virus fusion are G-protein-coupled chemokine receptors raises significant questions concerning the role of these signaling pathways in processes of virus entry, inhibition by β-chemokines, and pathogenesis. The convergence of diverse fields from HIV-1 research to chemotactic cytokines and their G-protein-coupled receptors would suggest that answers to these questions will be forthcoming.

Acknowledgement. This work was supported by Public Health Service grants 5-RO1-AI32393-04 (MLG), 5-RO1-AI29852-07 (KJW) and 5-P30-AI28662-08 (Duke CFAR) from the National Institutes of Health.

References

1. Albert J, Gaines H, Sonnerborg A, Nystrom G, Pehrson PO, Chiodi F, Sydow M von, Moberg L, Lidman K, Christensson B (1987) Isolation of human immunodeficiency virus (HIV) from plasma during primary HIV infection. J Med Virol 23:67
2. Baier M, Werner A, Bannert N, Metzner K, Kurth R (1995) HIV suppression by interleukin-16. Nature 378:563
3. Barker TD, Weissman D, Daucher JA, Roche KM, Fauci AS (1996) Identification of multiple and distinct CD8$^+$ T cell suppressor activites. J Immunol 156:4476
4. Barre-Sinoussi F, Chermann JC, Rey F, Nugeyre MT, Chamaret S, Gruest J, Dauguet C, Axler-Blin C, Vezinet-Brun F, Rouzioux C, Rozenbaum W, Montagnier L (1983) Isolation of a T lymphotropic retrovirus from a patient at risk for acquired immune deficiency syndrome (AIDS). Science 220:868
5. Biesinger B, Muller-Fleckenstein I, Simmer B, Lang G, Wittmann S, Platzer E, Desrosiers R, Fleckenstein B (1992) Stable growth transformation of human T lymphocytes by herpesvirus saimiri. Proc Natl Acad. Sci. USA 89:3116
6. Borrow P, Lewicki H, Hahn BH, Shaw GM, Oldstone MBA (1994) Virus-specific CD8$^+$ cytotoxic T lymphocyte activity associated with control of viremia in primary human immunodeficiency virus type 1 infection. J Virol 68:6103
7. Brinchmann JE, Gaudernack G, Thorsby E, Jonassen TO, Vartdal F (1989) Reliable isolation of human immunodeficiency virus from cultures of naturally infected CD4$^+$ cells. J Virol Methods 25:293
8. Brinchmann JE, Gaudernack G, Vartdal F (1990) CD8$^+$ T cells inhibit HIV replication in naturally infected CD4$^+$ cells. Evidence for a soluble inhibitor J Immunol 144:2961
9. Brinchmann JE, Gaudernack G, Vartdal F (1991) In vitro replication of HIV-1 in naturally infected CD4$^+$ T cells is inhibited by rIFN-α_2 and by a soluble factor secreted by activated CD8$^+$ T cells but not by rIFN-β, rIFN-γ, or by recombinant tumor necrosis factor-α. J Acquir Immune Defic Syndr 4:480
10. Buchbinder SP, Katz MH, Hessol NA, O'Malley PM, Holmberg SD (1994) Long-term HIV-1-infection without immunologic progression. J Acquir Immune Defic Syndr 8:1123
11. Cao Y, Qin L, Zhang L, Safrit J, Ho DD (1995) Virological and immunological characterization of long-term survivors of human immunodeficiency virus type 1 infection. N Engl J Med 332:201
12. Castro BA, Walker CM, Eichberg JW, and Levy JA (1991) Suppression of human immunodeficiency virus replication by CD8$^+$ cells from infected and uninfected chimpanzees. Cell Immunol 132:246

13. Chen CH, Weinhold KJ, Bartlett JA, Bolognesi DP, Greenberg ML (1993) CD8$^+$ T lymphocyte-mediated inhibition of HIV-1 long terminal repeat transcription: a novel antiviral mechanism. AIDS Res Hum Retrov 9:1079

14. Clark SJ, Saag MS, Decker WD, Campbell-Hill S, Roberson JL, Veldkamp PJ, Kappes JC, Hahn BH, Shaw GM (1991) High titers of cytopathic virus in plasma of patients with symptomatic primary HIV-1-infection N Engl J Med 324:954

15. Cocchi F, DeVico AL, Garzino-Demo A, Arya SK, Gallo RC, Lusso P (1995) Identification of RANTES, MIP-1α, and MIP-1β as the major HIV-suppressive factors produced by CD8$^+$ T cells. Science; 270:1811

16. Conlon K, Lloyd A, Chattopadhyay U, Lukas N, Kunkel S, Schall T, Taub D, Morimoto C, Osborne J, Oppenheim J, Young H, Kelvin D, Ortaldo J (1995) CD8$^+$ and CD45RA$^+$ human peripheral blood lymphocytes are potent sources of macrophage inflammatory protein-1α, interleukin-8 and RANTES. Eur J Immunol 25:751

17. Coombs RW, Collier AC, Allain J-P, Mikora B, Leuther M, Gjerset GF, Corey L (1989) Plasma viremia in human immunodeficiency virus infection. N Engl J Med 321:1626

18. Copeland KFT, McKay PJ, Rosenthal KL (1995) Suppression of activation of the human immunodefiency virus long terminal repeat by CD8$^+$ cells is not lentivirus specific. J Acquir Immune Defic Syndr Res Human Retroviruses 11:1321

19. Daar ES, Moudgil T, Meyer RD, Ho DD (1991) Transient high levels of viremia in patients with primary human immunodeficiency virus type 1 infection. N Engl J Med 324:961

20. Dalgleish AG, Beverly PCL, Clapham PR, Crawford DH, Greaves MF, Weiss RA (1984) The CD4 (T4) antigen is an essential component of the receptor for the AIDS retrovirus. Nature 312:763

21. Deng HK, Choe S, Ellmeier W, Liu R, Unutmaz D, Burkhart M, Marzio PD, Marmon S, Sutton RE, Hill CM, Davis C, Peiper SC, Schall TJ, Littman DR, Landau NR (1996) Identification of a major coreceptor for entry of primary isolates of HIV-1. Nature 381: 661

22. Dragic T, Litwin V, Allaway GP, Martin S, Huang Y, Nagashima KA, Cayanan C, Maddon PJ, Koup RA, Moore JP, Paxton WA (1996) HIV-1 entry into CD4$^+$ cells is mediated by the chemokine receptor C C CKR 5. Nature 381: 667

23. D'Souza MP, Mathieson BJ (1996) Early phases of HIV-1-infection: workshop summary. AIDS Res Hum Retrov 12: 1

24. Embretson J, Zupancic M, Ribas JL, Burke A, Racz P, Tenner-Racz K, Haase AT (1993) Massive covert infection of helper T lymphocytes and macrophages by HIV during the incubation period of AIDS. Nature 362:359

25. Ennen J, Findeklee H, Dittmar MT, Norley S, Ernst M, Kurth R (1994) CD8$^+$ T lymphocytes of African green monkeys secrete an immunodeficiency virus-suppressing lymphokine. Proc Nat Acad Sci USA 91:7207

26. Eyster ME, Ballard JO, Gail MH, Drummond JE, Goedert JJ (1989) Predictive markers for the acquired immunodeficiency syndrome (AIDS) in hemophiliacs: persistence of p24 antigen and low T4 cell count. Ann Intern Med 110:963

27. Feng Y, Broder CC, Kennedy PE, Berger EA (1996) HIV-1 entry co-factor: functional cDNA cloning of a seven-transmembrane, G protein-coupled receptor. Science; 272:872

28. Gallo RC, Salahuddin SZ, Popovic M, Shearer GM, Kaplan M, Haynes BF, Palker TJ, Redfield R, Oleske J, Safai B, White G, Foster P, Markham PD (1984) Frequent detection and isolation of cytopathic retroviruses (HTLV-III) from patients with AIDS and at risk for AIDS. Science 224:500

29. Gomez AM, Smaill FM, Rosenthal KL (1994) Inhibition of HIV replication by CD8$^+$ T cells correlates with CD4 counts and clinical stage of disease. Clin Exp Immunol 97:68

30. Ho DD, Moudgil T, Alam M (1989) Quantitation of human immunodeficiency virus type 1 in the blood of infected persons. N Engl J Med 321:1621

31. Hogervorst E, Jurriaans S, Wolf F de, Wijk A van, Wiersma A, Valk M, Roos M, Gemen B van, Coutinho R, Miedema F, Goudsmit J (1995) Predictors for non- and slow progression in human immunodeficiency virus (HIV) type 1 infection: low viral RNA copy numbers in serum and maintenance of high HIV-1 p24-specific but not V3-specific antibody levels. J Infect Dis 171:811

32. Hsueh FW, Walker CM, Blackbourn DJ, Levy JA (1994) Suppression of HIV replication by CD8$^+$ cell clones derived from HIV-infected and Uninfected individuals. Cell: Immunol. 159:271

33. Kannagi M, Chalifoux LV, Lord CI, Letvin NL (1988) Suppression of simian immunodeficiency virus replication in vitro by CD8$^+$ lymphocytes. J Immunol 140:2237

34. Kirchfoff F, Greenough TC, Brettler DB, Sullivan JL, Desrosiers RC (1995) Brief report: absence of intact nef sequences in a long-term survivor with nonprogressive HIV-1-infection. N Engl J Med 332:228
35. Klatzmann D, Champagne E, Chamaret S, Gruest J, Guetard D, Hercend T, Gluckman J-C, Montagnier L (1984) T-lymphocyte T4 molecule behaves as the receptor for human retrovirus LAV. Nature 312:767
36. Koup RA, Safrit JT, Cao Y, Andrews CA, McLeod G, Borkowsky W, Farthing C, Ho DD (1994) Temporal association of cellular immune responses with the initial control of viremia in primary human immunodeficiency virus type 1 syndrome. J Virol 68:4650
37. Lacey SF, Chen C-H, Weinhold KJ, Greenberg ML (1995) Suppression of HIV-1 replication by primary and transformed CD8 cells. AIDS Res Human Retroviruses 11[Suppl]:S133
38. Learmont J, Tindall B, Evans L, Cunningham A, Cunningham P, Wells J, Penny R, Kaldor J, Cooper DA (1992) Long-term symptomless HIV-1-infection in recipients of blood products from a single donor. Lancet 340:863
39. Levy JA, Hoffman AD, Kramer SM, Landis JA, Shimabukuro JM, Oshiro LS (1984) Isolation of lymphocytopathic retroviruses from San Francisco patients with AIDS. Science 225:840
40. Mackewicz CE, Ortega HW, Levy JA (1991) CD8 cell anti-HIV activity correlates with the clinical state of the infected individual. J Clin Invest 87:1462
41. Mackewicz CE, Ortega H, Levy JA (1994) Effect of cytokines on HIV replication in CD4$^+$ lymphocytes: lack of identity with the CD8$^+$ cell antiviral factor. Cell Immunol 153:329
42. Mackewicz CE, Blackbourn DJ, Levy JA (1995) CD8$^+$ T cells suppress humin immunodeficiency virus replication by inhibiting viral transcription. Proc Natl Acad Sci USA 92:2308
43. Maddon PJ, Dalgleish AG, McDougal JS, Clapham PR, Weiss RA, Axel R (1986) The T4 gene encodes the AIDS virus receptor and is expressed in the immune system and the brain. Cell 47:333
44. Mellors JW, Kingsley LA, Rinaldo CR Jr, Todd JA, Hoo BS, Kokka RP, Gupta P (1995) Quantitation of HIV-1 RNA in plasma predicts outcome after seroconversion. Ann Intern Med 122:573
45. Michael NL, Vahey M, Burke DS, Redfield RR (1992) Viral DNA and mRNA expression correlate with the stage of human immunodeficiency virus (HIV) type 1 infection in humans: evidence for viral replication in all stages of HIV disease. J Virol 66:310
46. Michael NL, Chang G, D'arcy LA, Ehrenberg PK, Mariani R, Busch MP, Birx DL, Schwartz DH (1995) Defective accessory genes in a human immunodeficiency virus type 1-infected long-term survivor lacking recoverable virus. J Virol 69:4228
47. Pantaleo G, Graziosi C, Demarest JF, Butini L, Montroni M, Fox CH, Orenstein JM, Kotler DP, Fauci AS (1993) HIV infection is active and progressive in lymphoid tissue during the clinically latent stage of disease. Nature 362:355
48. Pantaleo G, Graziosi C, and Fauci AS (1993) Mechanisms of disease: the immunopathogenesis of human immunodeficiency virus infection. N Engl J Med 328:327
49. Pantaleo G, Menzo S, Vaccarezza M, Graziosi C, Cohen O, Demarest J, Montefiori D, Orenstein J, Fox C, Schrager L, Margolick J, Buchbinder S, Giorgi J, Fauci A (1995) Studies in subjects with long-term nonprogressive human immunodeficiency virus infection. N Engl J Med 332:209
50. Patterson BK, Till M, Otto P, Goolsby C, Furtado MR, McBride LJ, Wolinsky SM (1993) Detection of HIV-1 DNA and messenger RNA in individual cells by PCR-driven in situ hybridization and flow cytometry. Science 260:976
51. Paxton WA, Martin SR, Tse D, O'brien TR, Skurnick J, VanDevanter NL, Padian N, Braun JF, Kotler DP, Wolinsky SM, Koup RA (1996) Relative resistance to HIV-1-infection of CD4 lymphocytes from persons who remain uninfected despite multiple high-risk sexual exposures. Nature Med 2:412
52. Piatak, Jr. M, Saag MS, Yang LC, Clark SJ, Kappes JC, Luk K-C, Hahn BH, Shaw GM, Lifson JD (1993) High levels of HIV-1 in plasma during all stages of infection determined by competitive PCR. Science 259:1749
53. Poli G, Fauci AS (1993) Cytokine modulation of HIV expression. Semin Immunol 5:304.1
54. Powell DJ, Bednarik DP, Folks TM, Jehuda-Cohen T, Villinger F, Sell KW, Ansari AA (1993) Inhibition of cellular activation of retroviral replication by CD8$^+$ T cell derived from non-human primates. Clin Exp Immunol 91:473
55. Saksela K, Stevens C, Rubinstein P, Baltimore D (1994) Human immunodeficiency virus type 1 mRNA expression in peripheral blood cells predicts disease progression independently of the numbers of CD4$^+$ lymphocytes Proc Natl Acad Sci USA 91:1104

56. Sheppard HW, Lang W, Ascher MS, Vittinghoff E, Winkelstein W (1993) The characterization of non-progressors: long-term HIV-1-infection with stable CD4+ T cell levels. J Acquir Immune Defic Syndr 7:1159
57. Tindall B, Cooper DA (1991) Primary HIV infection: host responses and intervention strategies. J Acquir Immune Defic Syndr 5:1
58. Toso JF, Chen C-H, Mohr JR, Piglia L, Oei C, Ferrari G, Greenberg ML, Weinhold KJ (1995) Oligoclonal CD8+ lymphocytes from asymptomatic HIV-infected individuals inhibit HIV-1 replication. J Infect Dis 172: (in press)
59. Tsubota H, Lord CI, Watkins DI, Morimoto C, Letvin NL (1989) A cytotoxic T lymphocyte inhibits acquired immunodeficiency syndrome virus replication in peripheral blood lymphocytes. J Exp Med 169:1421
60. Walker BD, Plata F (1990) Cytotoxic T lymphocytes against HIV. J Acquir Immune Defic Syndr 4:177
61. Walker CM, Levy JA (1989) A diffusible lymphokine produced by CD8+ T lymphocytes suppresses HIV replication. Immunology 66:628
62. Walker CM, Moody DJ, Stites DP, Levy JA (1986) CD8+ lymphocytes can control HIV infection in vitro by suppressing virus replication. Science 234:1563
63. Walker CM, Thomson-Honnebier GA, Hsueh FC, Erickson AL, Pan L, Levy JA (1991) CD8+ cells from HIV-1-infected individuals inhibit acute infection by human and primate immunodeficiency viruses. Cell Immunol 137:420
64. Walker CM, Erickson AL, Hsueh FC, Levy JA (1991) Inhibition of human immunodeficiency virus replication in acutely infected CD4+ cells by CD8+ cells involves a non-cytotoxic mechanism. J Virol 65:5921

Note added in proof. After submission of this manuscript three additional reports identifying CC CKR5 as a fusion cofactor for HIV-1 appeared within 1 week of references 21 and 22 in the text. They were Aikhatib et al (1996) Science 272: 1995; Doranz et al (1996) Cell 85: 1149; and Choe et al (1996) Cell 85: 1135

Role of complement and Fc receptors in the pathogenesis of HIV-1 infection

David C. Montefiori

Department of Surgery, Duke University Medical Center, P.O. Box 2926, Durham, NC 27710, USA

Introduction

The Fc portion of immunoglobulin is important for complement activation and for targeting antigens to complement receptors (CR) and Fc receptors (FcR) on the surface of many cell types. Interactions with complement, CR and FcR can play both beneficial and pathological roles during viral infection. Activation of the classical or alternative complement pathways by epitopes and antibodies on microbial surfaces generates cleavage fragments of early complement component C3 that deposit on microbial surfaces and act as opsonins [104, 125]. Further activation of the terminal complement pathway can lead to assembly of the C5b-9 membrane attack complex (MAC) that forms transmembrane channels and eventually kills many targeted microbes, including certain viruses [48]. Opsonized virus particles that are not destroyed by the MAC may go on to bind CR on a variety of cell types. CR-binding can have consequences such as infection enhancement, virus clearance through the mononuclear phagocytic system, virus trapping in lymphoid tissues and B cell activation. Infection enhancement or phagocytosis also occurs when immune-complexed virus engages FcR on monocytes and macrophages.

An understanding of how human immunodeficiency virus type 1 (HIV-1) interacts with the complement system and FcR is beginning to emerge, raising important questions about the immunopathogenic mechanisms of HIV-1. This article reviews what is known about the interactions of HIV-1 with complement and FcR and describes some of the consequences they could have for the virus and its host.

Antibody-independent complement activation by HIV-1

HIV-1 activates complement through the alternative [12, 93, 98] and classical [118, 143, 145] pathways independently of virus-specific antibodies. Antibody-independent complement activation by HIV-1 is mediated by epitopes on the surface gp120 and transmembrane gp41 of the virus [143, 153, 162]. Both viral envelope glycoproteins are synthesized as a common gp160 precursor [3, 169]. gp120 is bound loosely to the virus surface through a non-covalent interaction with gp41 [70], and a high-affinity interaction between gp120 and the HLA class II receptor, CD4, is critical for infection [24, 74].

One site for classical complement pathway activation has been localized to a cryptic epitope in the ectodomain of gp41 that becomes exposed after gp120-CD4 binding [30, 81, 163]. Classical pathway activation by gp120 is increased by mannan-binding protein (MBP) [44], a C-type lectin present in normal human serum [159] that is elevated in HIV-1-infected individuals [137]. Naturally occurring IgM against asialo-oligosaccharide is another normal product which sensitizes HIV-1 for classical complement pathway activation [174]. Additional epitopes and mechanisms for complement activation by gp120 and gp41 in the absence of antibody probably exist but remain to be identified.

Activation of the alternative complement pathway is increased by agents that remove terminal sialic acid residues from the HIV-1 envelope glycoproteins or prevent sialic acid from being added during viral glycoprotein synthesis [93, 98]. Other enveloped viruses, including herpes simplex virus, Sindbis virus and vesicular stomatitis virus, exhibit a similar phenomenon [49, 88, 142]. Glycoprotein carbohydrate moieties containing sialic acid as a terminal residue block complement activation by preserving the function of factor H, which negatively controls activation of the alternative complement pathway through the C3b, Bb convertase [33]. Sialylation of viral glycoproteins is governed by the glycosylation pattern of the host cell while individual glycosylation sites are dictated by amino acid sequence as encoded by the viral genome [68, 116]. Approximately 50% of the molecular mass of gp120 and gp41 is estimated to be carbohydrate [3] and only a portion of the carbohydrate moieties on these glycoproteins are sialylated when synthesized in Chinese-hamster ovary cells [90] or H9 cells [36]. Thus, complement activation by the HIV-1 can be determined genetically by the virus and the host cell, and is regulated in part by sialic acid content.

Antibody-dependent complement activation by HIV-1

As will be described in later sections of this review, complement activation by HIV-1 is significantly elevated in the presence of envelope-specific antibodies. IgM, the first immunoglobulin usually produced in response to microbial infection, is the most powerful complement-activating immunoglobulin [147] and might be part of the initial immune response to HIV-1 infection [134]. All four IgG subclasses also activate complement but most effective are IgG1 and IgG3 [133, 147], which are the dominant IgG subclasses induced in response to HIV-1 infection [18, 62, 64, 80, 152]. Human monoclonal antibodies of the IgG1 and IgG2 subclass that recognize specific epitopes in gp41 have been shown to produce complement-mediated, antibody-dependent enhancement (C'-ADE) of HIV-1 infection in vitro [122, 124]. This observation confirms the ability of these two subclasses of antibodies to activate complement when bound to the virus. Detection of C'-ADE at serum dilutions exceeding 1:10 000 [121] further indicates that small amounts of antibody can facilitate an interaction of HIV-1 with complement.

Two subclasses of IgA are found in human serum but neither appears capable of activating complement when bound to their corresponding antigen [128]. Conversely, sialylated carbohydrate moieties on the IgA molecule are able to block alternative complement pathway activation by native antigens and by antigen-bound IgG [105, 106]. This raises the possibility that alternative complement pathway activation by envelope-bound IgM or IgG will sometimes be prevented by sialylated carbohydrate moieties on gp120, gp41 or an IgA molecule. The sialylated moieties could lie adjacent to an IgM or IgG in the linear envelope sequence or could be introduced from a distance by envelope conformation. Thus, not all complement-activating antibodies on the virus surface will be capable of activating complement.

Mechanism of escape from complement-mediated viral lysis

Complement activation by cell-free HIV-1 and HIV-1-infected cells is adequate for opsonization by early C3 cleavage products [92] but is not sufficient for terminal pathway activation and complement-mediated lysis [7, 43, 175]. The mechanism by which HIV-1 evades the lytic action of homologous complement has been linked to the presence of one or more host cell proteins on the virus surface that prevent MAC formation [82, 99, 129, 132, 150]. These inhibitors belong to a group of complement regulatory proteins whose principal function is to protect normal human cells from nonspecific complement destruction [63, 72]. Complement regulatory proteins CR1 (CD35), membrane cofactor protein (MCP, CD46) and decay accelerating protein (DAF, CD55) prevent formation of the C5 convertases needed for C5 activation. CD59 is a late inhibitor of MAC formation which binds C9 and prevents self assembly of the C5b-C9 MAC complex (Fig. 1).

Expression of CD55 and CD59 on the surface of lymphocytes from HIV-1-infected individuals was shown to be diminished relative to control lymphocytes [76, 172]. The diminished expression of CD55 was associated with a heightened sensitivity to complement lysis [76], making it possible that HIV-1-induced down-regulation of complement control proteins serves as a partial mechanism of CD4+ lymphocyte depletion in infected individuals. Whether the diminished expression of complement regulatory proteins is due to direct infection of cells or indirect effects, such as altered cytokine production, is not known.

Several complement regulatory proteins are expressed on the surface of common human T cell lines used for HIV-1 synthesis in vitro [99]. Three of these complement regulatory proteins, CD46, CD55 and CD59, are found on the surface of HIV-1 and the related simian immunodeficiency virus (SIV) when the viruses are grown in T cell lines and peripheral blood mononuclear cells [82, 99, 129]. The proteins appear to be obtained by HIV-1 and SIV as the viruses assemble, bud and release from the surface of infected cells. A variety of other host cell proteins are also found on the surface of HIV-1 and SIV [4]. Evidence that virus-associated CD55 and CD59 are functional comes from the finding that partial complement-mediated lysis can be induced, as measured by release of internal antigens, when antibodies to CD55 or CD59 are incubated with cell-free HIV-1 [82, 129] and cells infected with HIV-1 [132]. It remains to be determined whether the lysis was sufficient to inactivate virus infectivity. A dominant role for any single complement regulatory protein in protecting infectious HIV-1 from complement-mediated inactivation also remains to be determined, and it is possible that multiple regulators must be blocked before HIV-1-infectivity is neutralized by complement. In addition to the membrane-bound inhibitors described above, soluble factor H may be another important inhibitor of complement lysis that deserves consideration [114, 150].

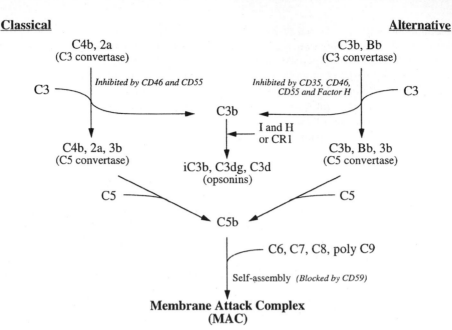

Fig. 1. Complement activation and membrane inhibitors of complement lysis. Classical and alternative pathways of complement activation generate C3 convertases, which cleave C3 to C3b on cell and virus surfaces. Factor I, in coordination with Factor H or complement receptor 1 (CR1), cleaves surface-bound C3b into iC3b and C3dg, which may be further cleaved to C3d. In addition to being an opsonin, C3b is an essential component of C5 convertases, which cleave C5 to C5b as the initial step in MAC self assembly. MAC formation is inhibited by CR1 (CD35), membrane cofactor protein (MCP; CD46), decay-accelerating protein (DAF; CD55) and Factor H, which prevent the formation of C5 convertases. CD59 is late inhibitor that prevents assembly of the C5b-C9 MAC complex by binding C9. Complement activation and its control elements are described in greater detail in several previous reviews [48, 104, 125]

Antibodies that block the function of one or more complement regulatory proteins on the virus surface might explain how xenoimmunized macaques were protected from SIV infection in early vaccine studies. Virus preparations used for immunization and subsequent challenge in those early studies were both grown in human cell lines, so it is not surprising that vaccine protection was attributed to the presence of antibodies to cellular proteins [22, 73]. We and others determined that anti-cell antibodies from these xenoimmunized macaques can render SIV and HIV-1 susceptible to complement-mediated lysis and inactivation [99, 146]. This would be expected if the anti-cell antibodies blocked the function of complement regulatory proteins on the virus surface, so that MAC formation could be induced by other antibodies. We found that plasmas from these animals did indeed contain antibodies to CD46 and CD59 [99]. Although reagents which selectively remove anti-CD46, anti-CD59 and antibodies to other complement regulatory proteins are needed to confirm their participation in SIV vaccine protection, these preliminary results led us to speculate that complement regulatory proteins might be suitable targets for alloimmunization and immunotherapy [91].

Complement-evasion strategies similar to that described above for HIV-1 and SIV are utilized by other viruses. Examples are the CD46-like activity of the 35-kDa secretory polypeptide encoded by vaccinia virus [69], and the CD55-like activity of envelope glycoprotein C of herpes simplex virus [35]. Another example is found in herpesvirus saimiri, which encodes a protein with structural and functional homology to CD59 [127]. HIV-1 and SIV appear to be unique in that they probably obtain complement regulatory proteins from the host rather than encoding them in their viral genome. By evading complement-mediated lysis, complement-opsonized HIV-1 particles are free to interact with complement receptors on a variety of cell types. As described below, some of these interactions have important implications for HIV-1-induced mechanisms of pathogenesis.

Infection enhancement

Complement activation in the absence of antibodies has been shown to enhance HIV-1-infection in a variety of cell types, including MT-2 cells [12, 93], U937 promonocytic cells [118, 144], Epstein-Barr virus (EBV)-transformed IC.1 B-cells [38] and Raji B cells [13]. This phenomenon also has been observed in THP-1 promonocytic cells and to a lesser degree in human peripheral blood monocytes, Mono Mac 6 monocytic cells and U251-MG glial cells [161]. Collectively, these studies determined that antibody-independent complement enhancement of HIV-1-infection in vitro can proceed through CR1, CR2 and CR3. Additional evidence suggests that complement and CR may sometimes permit HIV-1 to infect cells independently of CD4 [12, 13, 161].

Complement enhancement of HIV-1-infection is increased dramatically by envelope-specific antibody. C'-ADE of HIV-1-infection has several measurable effects in vitro, including a more rapid appearance of viral RNA, DNA, antigen and infectious virus particles [59, 121, 166]. C'-ADE has been detected with sera obtained at all stages of HIV-1-infection [95], including sera from long term non-progressors [102]. Detection of C'-ADE with sera from human volunteers immunized with gp160 [28, 61, 96], but not rgp120 (unpublished observation), is in agreement with reports that the dominant epitopes reside in two regions of gp41 corresponding to amino acids 586–620 and 644–663 of the gp160 molecule [122, 124]. Although the exact mechanism of C'-ADE is unknown, it appears to involve enhanced virus binding [6, 59, 97, 100] and internalization [6].

C'-ADE of HIV-1-infection has been observed in established cell lines of T cell (MT-2) and B cell (IC.1) origin, as well as in primary cultures of B lymphocytes and syncytiotrophoblasts (Table 1). Studies with complement component-deficient sera have determined that C'-ADE can utilize the alternative [120] and classical [59] pathways of complement activation. C'-ADE has a strict requirement for complement receptors and may utilize CR1 or CR2. Most studies have shown an additional requirement for CD4 (Table 1); one exception is a case where monoclonal antibody leu 3a to CD4 had very little impact on C'-ADE of HIV-1-infection in normal B lymphocytes [39]. Our inability to detect HIV-1 antigen in cultures of CR2+, CD4− Raji B cells for up to 8 weeks after virus exposure under conditions that favor C'-ADE [97] indicates that these conditions will not always lead to productive infection of CD4− cells. C'-ADE has also been reported for SIV, where the phenomenon parallels that of HIV-1 by requiring antibody, complement, CR2 and CD4 [94].

Measurements of C'-ADE that are made in established cell lines and with laboratory-adapted strains of HIV-1 do not necessarily predict natural antibody responses and have created doubts about their biological relevance [11]. Little effort has been made to evaluate C'-ADE as a correlate of HIV-1-induced immune suppres-

Table 1. Examples of complement-mediated antibody-dependent enhancement of HIV Infection

Cell type	HIV-1 strain	Activation pathway	CR utilized	CD4 required	Ref.
MT-2	IIIB, RF, primary isolates	Classical, alternative	CR2	Yes	[59, 102, 120, 123]
IC.1 B cells	LAV	nd	CR2	Yes	[38]
EBV-transformed B lymphocytes	IIIB and a primary isolate	nd	CR2	Yes	[166]
B lymphocytes	LAI	nd	CR1, CR2	No	[39]
Syncytiotrophoblasts	IIIB	nd	CR2	Yes	[165]

EBV, Epstein-Barr virus; CR, complement receptor; nd, not determined

sion using primary isolates and autologous sera. Studies in which complement was shown to enhance HIV-1-infection in cultures of normal B lymphocytes [39], thymocytes [26] and syncytiotrophoblasts [165], and where C'-ADE was observed with primary isolates [102, 166], may be taken as evidence that infection enhancement is operative to some extent in vivo. Subsets of normal CD4$^+$ lymphocytes that express low levels of CR1 [20] or CR2 [60] could be additional targets for C'-ADE of HIV-1-infection in vivo. One study showed a selective loss of CR2$^+$, CD4$^+$ lymphocytes in HIV-1-infected individuals [60], but it is not clear whether this loss was due to cell-killing or to down-regulation of CR2 expression on the cell surface [135]. Another study showed that gp120-antibody-complement complexes are present on the surface of uninfected lymphocytes from HIV-1-infected individuals, and it was suggested that this could be a mechanism by which the lymphocytes become targeted for immune elimination [25]; however, there is no indication that this has occurred in volunteers who received gp120 or gp160 subunit vaccines [37].

ADE of HIV-1-infection also may occur through FcR on monocytes and macrophages independently of complement (Table 2). Human monocytes and macrophages express three distinct classes of FcR for IgG, and one additional FcR for IgA. FcγRI and FcγRII are high- and low-affinity receptors, respectively, and are expressed on monocytes, macrophages and U937 human histiocytic lymphoma cells [117, 155]. FcγRIII is a low-affinity receptor that is expressed on macrophages and some T lymphocytes but is not found on monocytes or U937 cells [117, 155]. FcαR is expressed on monocytes, macrophages and some T lymphocytes [151].

FcR-ADE of HIV-1-infection has been observed in U937 cells and primary cultures of human lymphocytes, monocytes, macrophages and syncytiotrophoblasts, and has been shown to utilize FcγRI, FcγRIII and FcαR (Table 2). There is general agreement that FcR-ADE in U937 has a strict requirement for CD4 in addition to FcR, but CD4 may not be required in other cell types. Interestingly, CD4-independent FcR-ADE is observed when FcγRIII is utilized but not when cell surface FcγRIII expression is lacking, such as for U937 cells [155]. Epitopes for FcR-ADE of HIV-1-infection are present in the V3 loop of gp120 [66] and a conserved region of gp41 corresponding to amino acids 579–599 of gp160 [29]. In one study, FcR-ADE with patient isolates and autologous sera correlated with progression to disease in HIV-1-infected individuals [53].

Many examples exist of animal viruses that induce infection-enhancing antibodies, where the presence of these antibodies has been associated with higher levels of viremia, rapid disease progression, increased disease severity and vaccine failures [14,

Table 2. Examples of FcR-ADE of HIV Infection

Cell type	HIV strain	FcR utilized	CD4 required	Ref.
U937	IIIB	FcγRI	Yes	[57, 71, 75, 112, 154, 155, 176]
Lymphocytes	SF-128A, HIV-2/UC1, primary isolates	FcγRIII, other FcR	No	[52, 53]
Monocytes	IIIB	nd	nd	[75]
Macrophages	IIIB, Bal, SF-128A, HIV-2/UC1	FcγRIII,	Yes/No	[52, 112, 167]
Syncytiotrophoblasts	IIIB	FcγRIII, other FcR	No	[165]

nd, not determined

42, 115]. Lessons learned from these examples indicate that the in vivo manifestations of ADE are favored when viral variants arise that resist neutralization but remain sensitive to ADE in vitro. In this regard, HIV-1 exhibits extensive genetic variation throughout much of gp120 and gp41 [148] but less variation is seen in regions known to contain C′-ADE epitopes [122, 124]. Since it is common for neutralization-resistant variants of HIV-1 to appear during the course of infection [2], a newly arising HIV-1 variant to which no neutralizing antibody has been formed may be particularly susceptible to ADE [102]. These features of HIV-1 resemble viruses for which ADE is thought to produce clinically deleterious effects in vivo.

The ability to detect C′-ADE and FcR-ADE of HIV-1 infection in vitro using sera from vaccinated volunteers has raised concerns for HIV-1 vaccine development [14, 84]. Important examples of vaccine failures associated with ADE are found in equine infectious anemia virus (EIAV) and feline immunodeficiency virus (FIV), two viruses that belong to the same lentivirus family of retroviruses that includes HIV-1. Here, immunization with recombinant envelope subunit vaccines caused increased disease severity in ponies challenged with EIAV [170], and higher levels of virus replication in cats challenged with FIV [141]. It should be noted, however, that not all viruses that induce antibodies with ADE activity in vitro are subject to vaccine failure. Indeed, safe and effective vaccines exist for a number of viruses, including vaccines for yellow fever virus [160] and Japanese encephalitis virus [51]. These latter two viruses are important examples because both exhibit genetic variation and are known to induce antibodies capable of enhancing virus infection in vitro [14, 42, 115]. In addition, subunit vaccines and attenuated virus vaccines have protected macaques from SIV infection even though the vaccines induced antibodies with potent C′-ADE activity in vitro [101].

The pathological mechanisms which determine whether or not antibodies with ADE activity in vitro will produce deleterious clinical consequences and contribute to vaccine failure in vivo are unknown. Part of the problem in predicting these outcomes could be that our methods for detecting ADE in vitro are not an accurate representation of natural biological phenomena. This might explain why others have been unable to detect ADE of HIV-1-infection in cultures of normal human blood monocytes and peritoneal macrophages [139]. Another possibility is that the impact of ADE in the infected host is diminished when overriding protective immune responses are generated. The study of ADE in viral pathogenesis is, therefore, technically difficult and very complex but important to pursue.

Virus clearance

In contrast to the pathological implications associated with C′-ADE, complement activation by HIV-1 may in some ways be beneficial to the host. One example is found in the interaction of complement-opsonized particles with CR1. In addition to being a cofactor for the factor I-mediated cleavage of C3b to iC3b and C3dg, CR1 is a receptor for particulate antigens coated with C3b and iC3b C3 and is found on red blood cells (RBC), follicular dendritic cells (FDC), monocytes, macrophages, neutrophils, eosinophils, B lymphocytes and glomerular podocytes [104, 125]. RBC account for 90–95% of CR1 in the circulation, where it assists in transporting circulating immune complexes to the liver and spleen for destruction by fixed macrophages [126, 130].

Studies have shown that HIV-1 is produced continuously at high rates and rapidly cleared from circulation, where the plasma half-life is approximately 2 days and the turnover rate is approximately 6.8×10^8 plasma virions per day [50, 171]. More recent estimates place these rates at an even higher level [111]. Much of this clearance could be mediated through the mononuclear phagocytic system as aided by immune complex formation and subsequent trapping by CR1 on RBC. Envelope-specific antibodies and complement have been shown to target HIV-1 to CR1 on cell surfaces, including human RBC [100], increasing the likelihood that complement-activating antibodies facilitate HIV-1 immune complex clearance much the same as they clear other particulate antigens from the circulation. In addition to controlling plasma viremia during chronic infection, the initial reduction in plasma viremia that often follows primary HIV-1 infection [19, 23] might be governed in part by the first IgM and IgG antibodies generated by infection and that induce HIV-1 immune complex formation with complement.

High-affinity, multivalent interactions with FcR can lead to phagocytosis [32] as another mechanism by which HIV-1 could be cleared from circulation. Studies have shown that endocytosis through FcγRI, II and III on primary cultures of monocyte-derived macrophages can neutralize HIV-1-infectivity through intracellular lysozomal degradation [21, 79]. This mode of entry is different from the pH-independent process by which HIV-1 enters cells in the absence of antibody [86, 149]. The fact that FcR-ADE usually requires the use of highly diluted sera suggests that low concentrations of antibodies stabilize the virus on the cell surface through weak interactions with FcR to enhance infection, whereas higher antibody concentrations produce high-affinity, multivalent interactions with FcR needed for virus degradation [21, 79]. Hence, the fate of HIV-1 immune complexes that engage FcR might be determined in part by the quality and quantity of virus-specific antibody induced by infection.

Virus trapping in lymphoid tissues

Extracellular trapping of HIV-1 on the surface of FDC creates a major reservoir of the virus in lymphoid tissues. It has been suggested that this reservoir serves as a source of antigen in generating and maintaining immune responses, and also serves as a source of virus to be transferred to CD4+ cells for infection [45, 108, 109]. Virus trapping on FDC most likely depends on antibody and complement. FDC express a high density of CR1, CR2 and CR3 on the cell surface [119], and account for the majority of C3-dependent antigen retention in lymphoid tissues [65]. In this regard, HIV-1 trapping on human tonsillar FDC in vitro was shown to be dependent on C3 activation and to be increased by antibodies from infected individuals [56]. Antibodies and complement could impart infection-enhancing properties on the trapped virus and, although this does not permit infection of FDC prior to the onset of AIDS [131], it might explain why HIV-1 immune complexes on the surface of tonsillar FDC were transferable and infectious for CD4+ lymphocytes even when coated with neutralizing antibodies [45].

B cell abnormalities

A requirement for CR in the detection of C'-ADE of HIV-1 infection [123, 166] indicates that opsonized virus particles bind the complement ligation site on CR, and we confirmed this for CR2 on Raji-3 and MT-2 cells [97]. CR2 is a 145-kDa transmembrane glycoprotein that is expressed in high abundance on B lymphocytes and is a receptor for Epstein-Barr virus and for the C3 cleavage products, C3dg and C3d [1]. CR2 is expressed on immature and mature B cells and disappears when the cells are actively proliferating or when terminally differentiated into plasma cells [157].

Multivalent ligation of CR2 on B lymphocytes is known to cooperate with membrane IgM to elicit a calcium-dependent signal transduction mechanism [17, 85, 168] and to cause B cell activation and proliferation [10, 15, 89, 173]. Activation is triggered when cross-linked CR2 engages a CD19-containing complex of proteins on the B cell surface [85] and is accompanied by increased c-fos mRNA levels [78]. In view of these observations, HIV-1-infection is associated with a number of B cell abnormalities, including polyclonal B cell activation [83, 140] and an increased incidence of B cell lymphoma [9, 138]. A possible role for HIV-1 immune complexes in inducing these abnormalities has been largely ignored. Studies are needed to determine whether cellular activation signals induced by the multivalent ligation of complement-opsonized HIV-1 with CR2 is a process leading to polyclonal B cell activation. It also seems possible that constant B cell stimulation through CR2 during chronic HIV-1-infection would eventually lead to neoplastic transformation. In addition to these positive signalling mechanisms, down-regulation of CR2 on B cells during HIV-1-infection [135] might impair normal B cell responsiveness. Future studies that focus on CR2 effector mechanisms might provide insights into this aspect of HIV-1 pathogenesis.

CR2-ligand interactions in the control of immune responses

CR2 and its complement ligands have been linked to the induction of antigen-driven primary antibody responses to T-dependent and T-independent antigens [16, 46, 47, 164], including the generation of memory B cells [65]. Part of this activity is associated with the long-term retention of antigen in the form of non-degraded immune complexes on the surface of FDC [158]. Germinal centers of lymphoid organs are sites of antigen-driven B cell proliferation, somatic mutation, positive and negative selection, and memory B cell development [55, 77]. Non-recirculating B cells that express CR2 can transport immune complexes to FDC where the immune complexes are retained and participate in T cell-dependent responses [31, 40]. Cell signaling mechanisms associated with membrane IgM and CR2 cross-linking on B lymphocytes also may cooperate to generate antibody responses [5, 16, 41, 85, 168].

Support for a role of CR2 in the induction of antibody responses comes from a recent study in which the threshold concentration of antigen required to induce an antibody response in mice was reduced by as much as 100-fold by fusing the antigen to C3d for delivery to CR2 [27]. One can envision how C3d-coated HIV-1 particles would be delivered to B lymphocytes through multivalent interactions with CR2 to enhance the initial immune response to infection. High levels of plasma virus produced during the acute stage of primary infection [19, 23] might begin this process through complement-activating epitopes on gp120 and gp41 prior to antibody production. The first IgM and IgG antibodies to appear would increase the level of C3d deposition on the virus, thereby continuing to drive the developing antibody response. In this regard, factors controlling complement activation by HIV-1, such as host cell glycosylation patterns, and epitopes for complement activation and complement-activating antibodies on the virus surface, could be important determinants of the initial antibody response to infection. Support for this model will require studies of complement activation, immunoglobulin class and subclass production, and virus opsonization during the first few weeks to months of primary HIV-1-infection.

Complement and FcR in HIV-1-infected individuals

Multiple lines of evidence indicate that complement is chronically activated in HIV-1-infected individuals [113, 136]. Part of this activation may be driven by epitopes and antibodies on the envelope glycoproteins of cell-free virus and on the surface of infected cells. The observation that immune complexes isolated from the plasma of HIV-1-infected individuals contain complement, antibody, viral p24 core protein and infectious virus [34, 67, 87, 103, 107] confirms that HIV-1 activates complement in vivo. In one study, polyethylene glycol-precipitable HIV-1 immune complexes in sera from infected individuals exhibited properties that resembled FcR-ADE when used to infect U937 cells [67].

It is not known how early in HIV-1-infection the complement cascade becomes activated. Studies performed during acute primary HIV-1-infection are needed to determine whether complement-activating antibodies contribute to the initial reduction in plasma viremia by facilitating virus clearance through the mononuclear phagocytic system, by inducing viral lysis or by redistributing the virus to other compartments.

Individuals in late stages of HIV-1-infection have a decreased density of CR1 on their RBC and an increase in circulating immune complexes [8, 54, 58, 156]. The increase in circulating immune complexes might be explained by defective clearance owing to the low density of CR1 on their RBC. Impaired FcR functions might further contribute to defective immune complex clearance during advanced stages HIV-1-infection [8]. Without these normal functions of the mononuclear phagocytic system, uncontrolled levels of circulating immune complexes are likely to contribute to immune suppression and, by accumulating in vessel walls, produce other pathological conditions, such as AIDS-associated glomerulitis [110].

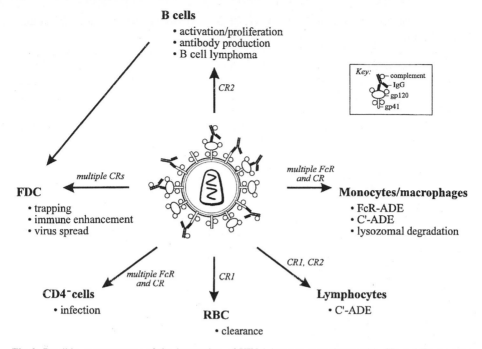

Fig. 2. Possible consequences of the interaction of HIV-1 immune complexes with CR and Fc receptor (FcR). Activated fragments of complement component C3 are deposited on the virus surface as a result of complement activation by epitopes and the Fc portion of antibodies on gp120 and gp41. Complement deposition may target the virus to: (1) multiple CR on CD4$^+$ lymphocytes, monocytes and macrophages for enhanced infection, (2) CR1 on red blood cells (RBC) for virus clearance through the mononuclear phagocytic system, (3) multiple CR on follicular dendritic cells (FDC) for virus trapping in lymphoid tissues and (4) CR2 on B lymphocytes for cellular activation, enhanced antibody production, possible neoplastic transformation and transportation of HIV-1 immune complexes to lymphoid tissues for entrapment on FDC. The Fc portion of antibodies bound to the virus surface may target the virus to FcR on monocytes and macrophages where: (1) low-affinity interactions lead to infection-enhancement and (2) high-affinity, multivalent interactions lead to lysozomal degradation. FcR binding may cooperate with CR binding in either of these latter processes. Independent or cooperative binding to CR and FcR may also permit infection of certain CD4$^-$ cell types. Not shown on the virus surface surface are cellular proteins, including the complement regulatory proteins CD46, CD55, CD59 and Factor H

Conclusions

HIV-1 clearly utilizes a variety of antibody-dependent and -independent mechanisms for complement activation and opsonization, while at the same time it possesses the means to evade MAC destruction. Such an efficient mode of complement utilization is an indication that the virus must be coated with complement to ensure its survival. Possible advantages afforded by complement are: (1) to facilitate virus entry for infection, (2) to trap virus on the surface of FDC, thereby creating a reservoir of infectious virus to be transferred to infection-susceptible cells, and (3) to disrupt normal B cell functions in evading immune surveillance. Complement activation, however, comes at some cost to the virus, since it may facilitate virus clearance through the mononuclear phagocytic system and enhance the immunogenicity of viral antigens. In addition, antibodies that target the virus to FcR on monocytes and macrophages might enhance virus infection under conditions of low-affinity FcR engagement, or neutralize the virus by lysozomal degradation under conditions of high-affinity, multivalent FcR engagement.

A balance in the milieu of HIV-1 interactions with complement and FcR could be one of the many factors that keep virus replication in equilibrium with its host for a period of clinical latency while maintaining viral persistence. Disturbing the normal balance of interactions between HIV-1, complement and FcR could possibly delay or accelerate progression to disease. The balance may be disturbed by genetic variation in viral glycosylation sites, different glycosylation patterns of various host cells, changes in antibody specificity, class and subclass, and altered cell surface expression of CR, FcR and complement regulatory proteins. Some of these changes could be brought on by direct infection of cells or by secondary effects of infection, such as abnormal cytokine production and co-infection with other agents.

Acknowledgements. The author thanks Dr. Dani P. Bolognesi for his critical review of the manuscript, Susan Hellenbrand for her assistance in designing figures and Thomas Lore for his aid in preparing the manuscript.

References

1. Ahearn JM, Fearon DT (1989) Structure and function of the complement receptors, CR1 (CD35) and CR2 (CD21). Adv Immunol 46:183
2. Albert J, Abrahamsson B, Nagy K, Aurelius E, Gaines H, Nystrom G, Fenyo EM (1990) Rapid development of isolate-specific neutralizing antibodies after primary HIV-1-infection and consequent emergence of virus variants which resist neutralization by autologous sera. J Acquir Immune Defic Syndr 4:107
3. Allan JS, Coligan JE, Barin F, McLane MF, Sodroski JG, Rosen CA, Haseltine WA, Lee TH, Essex M (1985) Major glycoprotein antigens that induce antibodies in AIDS patients are encoded by HTLV-III. Science 228:1091
4. Arthur LO, Bess JW, Sowder RC, Benveniste RE, Mann DL, Chermann J-C, Henderson LE (1991) Cellular proteins bound to immunodeficiency viruses: implications for pathogenesis and vaccines. Science 258:1935
5. Ashwell JD (1988) Are B lymphocytes the principal antigen-presenting cells in vivo? J Immunol 140:3697
6. Bakker LJ, Nottet HSLM, Vos NM de, Graaf L de, Strijp JAG van, Visser MR, Verhoef J (1992) Antibodies and complement enhance binding and uptake of HIV-1 by human monocytes. J Acquir Immune Defic Syndr 6:35
7. Banapour B, Sernatinger J, Levy JA (1986) The AIDS-associated retrovirus is not sensitive to lysis or inactivation by human serum. Virology 152:268
8. Bender BS, Davidson BL, Kline R, Brown C, Quinn TC (1988) Role of the mononuclear phagocytic system in the immunopathogenesis of human immunodeficiency virus infection and the acquired immunodeficiency syndrome. Rev Infect Dis 10:1142
9. Beral V, Peterman T, Berkelman R, Jaffe H (1991) AIDS-associated non-Hodgkin lymphoma. Lancet 337:805
10. Bohnsack JF, Cooper NR (1988) CR2 ligands modulate human B cell activation. J Immunol 141:2569
11. Bolognesi DP (1989) Do antibodies enhance the infection of cells by HIV? Nature 340:431
12. Boyer V, Desgranges C, Trabaud M-A, Fischer E, Kazatchkine MD (1991) Complement mediates human immunodeficiency virus type 1 infection of a human T cell line in a CD4$^-$ and antibody-independent fashion. J Exp Med 173:1151
13. Boyer V, Delibrias C, Noraz N, Fischer E, Kazatchkine MD, Desgranges C (1992) Complement receptor type 2 mediates infection of the human CD4-negative Raji B-cell line with opsonized HIV. Scan J Immunol 36:879
14. Burke SB (1992) Human HIV vaccine trials: does antibody-dependent enhancement pose a genuine risk? Perspect Biol Med 35:511

15. Carter RH, Fearon DT (1989) Polymeric C3dg primes human lymphocytes for proliferation induced by anti-IgM. J Immunol 143:1755
16. Carter RH, Fearon DT (1992) CD19: lowering the threshold for antigen receptor stimulation of B lymphocytes. Science 256:105
17. Carter RH, Spycher MO, Ng YC, Hoffman R, Fearon DT (1988) Synergistic interaction between complement receptor type 2 and membrane IgM on B lymphocytes. J Immunol 141:457
18. Chiodi F, Mathiesen T, Albert J, Parks E, Norrby E, Wahren B (1989) IgG subclass responses to a transmembrane protein (gp41) peptide in HIV infection. J Immunol 142:3809
19. Clark SJ, Saag MS, Decke WD, Campbell-Hill S, Roberson JL, Veldkamp PJ, Kappes JC, Hahn BH, Shaw GM (1991) High titers of cytopathic virus in plasma of patients with symptomatic primary HIV-1 infection. N Engl J Med 324:954
20. Cohen JHM, Aubry JP, Revillard JP, Banchereau J, Kazatchkine MD (1989) Human T lymphocytes expressing the C3b/C4b complement receptor type one (CR1, CD35) belong to Fcγ receptor-positive CD4-positive T cells. Cell Immunol 121:383
21. Connor RI, Dinces NB, Howell AL, Romet-Lemonne J-L, Pasquali J-L, Fanger MW (1991) Fc receptors for IgG (FcγRs) on human monocytes and macrophages are not infectivity receptors for human immunodeficiency virus type 1 (HIV-1): studies using bispecific antibodies to target HIV-1 to various myeloid cell surface molecules, including FcγR. Proc Natl Acad Sci USA 88:9593
22. Cranage MP, Polyanskaya N, McBride B, Cook N, Ashworth LAE, Dennis M, Baskerville A, Greenaway PJ, Corcoran T, Kitchen P, Rose J, Murphey-Corb M, Desrosiers RC, Stott EJ, Farrar GH (1993) Studies on the specificity of the vaccine effect elicited by inactivated simian immunodeficiency virus. AIDS Res Hum Retroviruses 9:13
23. Daar ES, Moudgil T, Meyer RD, Ho DD (1991) Transient high levels of viremia in patients with primary human immunodeficiency virus type 1 infection. N Engl J Med 324:961
24. Dalgleish AG, Beverley PCL, Clapham PR, Crawford DH, Greaves MF, Weiss RA (1984) The CD4 (T4) antigen is an essential component of the receptor for the AIDS retrovirus. Nature 312:763
25. Daniel V, Susal C, Weimer R, Zimmerman R, Huth-Kuhne A, Opelz G (1993) Association of T cell and macrophage dysfunction with surface gp120 immunoglobulin-complement complexes in HIV-infected patients. Clin Exp Med 93:152
26. Delibrias C-C, Mouhoub A, Fischer E, Kazatchkine MD (1994) CR1 (CD35) and CR2 (CD21) complement C3 receptors are expressed on normal human thymocytes and mediate infection of thymocytes with opsonized human immunodeficiency virus. Eur J Immunol 24:2784
27. Dempsey PW, Allison MED, Akkaraju S, Goodnow CC, Fearon DT (1996) C3d of complement as a molecular adjuvant: bridging innate and acquired immunity. Science 271:348
28. Dolin R, Graham BS, Greenberg SB, Tacket CO, Belshe RB, Midthun K, Clements ML, Gorse GJ, Horgan BW, Atmar RL, Karzon DT, Bonnez W, Fernie BF, Montefiori DC, Stablien DM, Smith GE, Koff WC, the NIAID AIDS Vaccine Clinical Trials Network (1991) The safety and immunogenicity of a human immunodeficiency virus type 1 (HIV-1) recombinant gp160 candidate vaccine in humans. Ann Intern Med 114:119
29. Eaton AM, Ugen KE, Weiner DB, Wildes T, Levy JA (1994) An anti-gp41 human monoclonal antibody that enhances HIV-1 infection in the absence of complement. AIDS Res Hum Retroviruses 10:13
30. Ebenbichler CF, Thielens NM, Vornhagen R, Marschang P, Arlaud GJ, Dierich MP (1991) Human immunodeficiency virus type 1 activates the classical pathway of complement by direct C1 binding through specific sites in the transmembrane glycoprotein gp41. J Exp Med 174:1417
31. Erdie A, Fust G, Gergely J (1991) The role of C3 in the immune response. Immunol Today 12:332
32. Fanger MW, Shen L, Graziano RF, Guyre PM (1989) Cytotoxicity mediated by human Fc receptors for IgG. Immunol Today 10:92
33. Fearon DT (1978) Regulation of membrane sialic acid of B1H-dependent decay dissociation of amplification C3 convertase of the alternative complement pathway. Proc Natl Acad Sci USA 75:1971
34. Fiscus SA, Folds JD, Horst CM van der (1993) Infectious immune complexes in HIV-1-infected patients. Viral Immunol 6:135
35. Fries LF, Friedman HM, Cohen GH, Eisenberg RJ, Hammer CH, Frank MM (1986) Glycoprotein C of Herpes simplex virus type 1 is an inhibitor of the complement cascade. J Immunol 137:1636
36. Geyer H, Holschbach C, Hunsman C, Schneider J (1988) Carbohydrates of human immunodeficiency virus: structures of oligosaccharides linked to the envelope glycoprotein gp120. J Biol Chem 263:11760

37. Graham, BS, Wright PF (1995) Candidate AIDS Vaccines. N Engl J Med 333:1331
38. Gras GS, Dormont D (1991) Antibody-dependent and antibody-independent complement-mediated enhancement of human immunodeficiency virus type 1 infection in a human, Epstein-Barr virus-transformed B-lymphocytic cell line. J Virol 65:541
39. Gras G, Richard Y, Roques P, Olivier R, Dormont D (1993) Complement and virus-specific antibody-dependent infection of normal B lymphocytes by human immunodeficiency virus type 1. Blood 81:1808
40. Gray D, Skarvall H (1988) B-cell memory is short-lived in the absence of antigen. Nature 336:70
41. Grosjean I, Lachaux A, Bella C, Aubry J-P, Bonnefoy J-V, Kaiserlian D (1994) CD23/CD21 interaction is required for presentation of soluble protein antigen by lymphoblastoid B cell lines to specific CD4+ T cell clones. Eur J Immunol 24:2982
42. Halstead SB (1982) Immune enhancement of viral infection. Prog Allergy 31:301
43. Harada S, Yoshiyama H, Yamamoto N (1985) Effect of heat and fresh human serum on the infectivity of human T cell lymphotropic virus type III evaluated with new bioassay systems. J Clin Microbiol 22:908
44. Haurum JS, Thiel S, Jones IM, Fischer PB, Laursen SB, Jensenius JC (1993) Complement activation upon binding of mannan-binding protein to HIV envelope glycoproteins. J Acquir Immune Defic Syndr 7:1307
45. Heath SL, Tew JG, Tew JG, Szakal AK, Burton GF (1995) Follicular dendritic cells and human immunodeficiency virus infectivity. Nature 377:740
46. Hebell T, Ahearn JM, Fearon DT (1991) Suppression of the immune response by a soluble complement receptor of B lymphocytes. Science 254:102
47. Heyman B, Wiersma EJ, Kinoshita T (1991) In vivo inhibition of the antibody response by a complement receptor-specific monoclonal antibody. J Exp Med 172:665
48. Hirsch RL (1982) The complement system: its importance in the host response to viral infection. Microbiol Rev 46:71
49. Hirsch RL, Wolinsky JS, Winkelstein JA (1986) Activation of the alternative complement pathway by mumps infected cells: relationship to viral neuraminidase activity. Arch Virol 87:181
50. Ho DD, Neumann AU, Perelson AS, Chen W, Leonard JM, Markowitz M (1995) Rapid turnover of plasma virions and CD4 lymphocytes in HIV-1-infection. Nature 373:123
51. Hoke CH, Nisalak A, Sangawhipa N, Jatanasen S, Laorakapongse T, Innis BL, Kotchasenee S-O, Gingrich JB, Latendresse J, Fukai K, Burke DS (1988) Protection against japanese encephalitis by inactivated vaccines. N Engl J Med 319:608
52. Homsy J, Meyer M, Tateno M, Clarkson S, Levy JA (1989) The Fc and not CD4 receptor mediates antibody enhancement of HIV infection in human cells. Science 244:1357
53. Homsy J, Meyer M, Levy JA (1990) Serum enhancement of human immunodeficiency virus (HIV) infection correlates with disease in HIV-infected individuals. J Virol 64:1437
54. Inada Y, Lange M, McKinley GF, Sonnabend JA, Fonville TW, Kanemitsu T, Tanaka M, Clark WS (1986) Hematologic correlates and the role of erythrocyte CR1 (C3b receptors) in the development of AIDS. AIDS Res 2:235
55. Jacob J, Kelsoe G, Rajewsky K, Weiss U (1991) Intraclonal generation of antibody mutants in germinal centres. Nature 354:389
56. Joling P, Bakker LJ, Van Strijp JAG, Meerloo T, Graaf L de, Dekker MEM, Goudsmit J, Verhoef J, Schuurman H-J (1993) Binding of human immunodeficiency virus type-1 to follicular dendritic cells in vitro is complement dependent. J Immunol 150:1065
57. Jouault T, Chapuis F, Olivier R, Parravicini C, Bahraoui E, Gluckman J-C (1989) HIV infection of monocytic cells: role of antibody-mediated virus binding to Fcγ receptors. AIDS 3:125
58. Jouvin M-H, Rozenbaum W, Russo R, Kazatchkine MD (1987) Decreased expression of the C3b/C4b complement receptor (CR1) in AIDS and AIDS-related syndromes correlates with clinical subpopulations of patients with HIV infection. J Acquir Immune Defic Syndr 1:89
59. June RA, Schade SZ, Bankowski MJ, Kuhns M, McNamara A, Lint TF, Landay AL, Spear GT (1991) Complement and antibody mediate enhancement of HIV infection by increasing virus binding and provirus formation. J Acquir Immune Defic Syndr 5:269
60. June RA, Landay AL, Stefanik K, Lint TF, Spear GT (1992) Phenotypic analysis of complement receptor 2+ T lymphocytes: reduced expression on CD4+ cells in HIV-infected persons. Immunology 75:59

61. Keefer MC, Graham BS, Belshe RB, Schwartz D, Corey L, Bolognesi DP, Stablein DM, Montefiori DC, McElrath J, Clements ML, Gorse GJ, Wright PF, Matthews TJ, Smith GE, Lawrence D, Dolin R, the NIAID AIDS Vaccine Clinical Trials Network (1994) Studies of high doses of a human immunodeficiency virus type 1 (HIV-1) recombinant gp160 candidate vaccine in HIV-1 seronegative humans. AIDS Res Hum Retroviruses 10:1713

62. Khalife J, Guy B, Capron M, Kieny M-P, Ameisen J-C, Montagnier L, Lecocq J-P, Capron A (1988) Isotypic restriction of antibody response to human immunodeficiency virus. AIDS Res Hum Retroviruses 4:3

63. Kinoshita T (1991) Biology of complement: the overture. Immunol Today 12:291

64. Klasse PJ, Blomberg J (1987) Patterns of antibodies to human immunodeficiency virus proteins in different subclasses of IgG. J Infect Dis 156:1026

65. Klaus GGB, Humphrey JH, Kunkle A, Dongworth DW (1980) The follicular dendritic cell: its role in antigen presentation in the generation of immunological memory. Immunol Rev 53:3

66. Kliks SC, Shioda T, Haigwood NL, Levy JA (1993) V3 variability can influence the ability of an antibody to neutralize or enhance infection by diverse strains of human immunodeficiency virus type 1. Proc Natl Acad Sci USA 90:11518

67. Kobayashi K, Takeda A, Green S, Tuazon CU, Ennis FA (1993) Direct detection of infectious human immunodeficiency virus type 1 (HIV-1) immune complexes in the sera of HIV-1-infected persons. J Infect Dis 168:729

68. Kornfeld R, Kornfeld S (1985) Assembly of asparagine-linked oligosaccharides. Annu Rev Biochem 54:631

69. Kotwal GJ, Isaacs SN, McKenzie R, Frank MM, Moss B (1990) Inhibition of the complement cascade by the major secretory protein of vaccinia virus. Science 250:827

70. Kowalski M, Potz J, Basiripour L, Dorfman T, Goh WC, Terwilliger E, Dayton A, Rosen C, Haseltine W, Sodroski J (1987) Functional regions of the envelope glycoprotein of human immunodeficiency virus type 1. Science 237:1351

71. Kozlowski PA, Black KP, Shen L, Jackson S (1995) High prevalence of serum IgA HIV-1-infection-enhancing antibodies in HIV-infected persons. J Immunol 154:6163

72. Lachman PJ (1991) The control of homologous lysis. Immunol Today 12:312

73. Langlois AJ, Weinhold KJ, Matthews TJ, Greenberg ML, Bolognesi DP (1992) Detection of anti-human cell antibodies in sera from macaques immunized with whole inactivated virus. AIDS Res Hum Retroviruses 8:1641

74. Lasky LA, Nakamura G, Smith DH, Fennie C, Shimasaki C, Patzer E, Berman P, Gregory T, Capon DJ (1987) Delineation of a region of the human immunodeficiency virus gp120 glycoprotein critical for interaction with the CD4 receptor. Cell 50:975

75. Laurence J, Saunders A, Early E, Salmon JE (1990) Human immunodeficiency virus infection of monocytes: relationship to Fcγ receptors and antibody-dependent viral enhancement. Immunol 70:338

76. Lederman MM, Purvis SF, Walter EI, Carey JT, Medof ME (1989) Heightened complement sensitivity of acquired immunodeficiency syndrome lymphocytes related to diminished expression of decay-acelerating factor. Proc Natl Acad Sci USA 86:4205

77. Liu Y-J, Johnson GD, Gordon J, MacLennan ICM (1992) Germinal centres in T cell-dependent antibody responses. Immunol Today 13:17

78. Luxembourg AT, Cooper NR (1994) Modulation of signaling via the B cell antigen receptor by CD21, the receptor for C3dg and EBV. J Immunol 153:4448

79. Mabondzo A, Aussage P, Bartholeyns J, Le Naour R, Raoul H, Romet-Lemonne J-L, Dormont D (1992) Bispecific antibody targeting of human immunodeficiency virus type 1 (HIV-1) glycoprotein 41 to human macrophages through the Fc IgG receptor I mediates neutralizing effects in HIV-1-infection. J Infect Dis 166:93

80. Mann DL, Hamlin-Green G, Willoughby A, Landesman SH, Goedert, JJ (1994) Immunoglobulin class and subclass antibodies to HIV proteins in maternal serum: association with perinatal transmission. J Acquir Immune Defic Syndr 7:617

81. Marschang P, Gurtler L, Totsch M, Thielens NM, Arlaud GJ, Hittmair A, Katinger H, Dierich MP (1993) HIV-1 and HIV-2 isolates differ in their ability to activate the complement system on the surface of infected cells. J Acquir Immune Defic Syndr 7:903

82. Marschang P, Sodroski J, Wurzner R, Dierich MP (1995) Decay-accelerating factor (CD55) protects human immunodeficiency virus type 1 from inactivation by human complement. Eur J Immunol 25:285

83. Martinez-Maza O, Crabb E, Mitsuyasu RT, Fahey JL, Giorgi JV (1987) Infection with the human immunodeficiency virus (HIV) is associated with an in vivo increase in B lymphocyte activation and immaturity. J Immunol 138:3720

84. Mascola JR, Matthieson BJ, Zack PM, Walker MC, Halstead SB, Burke DS (1993) Summary report: workshop on the potential risks of antibody-dependent enhancement in human HIV vaccine trials. AIDS Res Hum Retroviruses 9:1175

85. Matsumoto AK, Kopicky-Burd J, Carter RH, Tuveson DA, Tedder TF, Fearon DT (1991) Intersection of the complement and immune systems: a signal transduction complex of the B lymphocyte-containing complement receptor type 2 and CD19. J Exp Med 173:55

86. McClure MO, Marsh M, Weiss RA (1987) Human immunodeficiency virus type 1 infection of CD4-bearing cells occurs by a pH-independent mechanism. EMBO J 7:513

87. McHugh TM, Stites DP, Busch MP, Krowka JF, Stricker RB, Hollander H (1988) Relation of circulating levels of human immunodeficiency virus (HIV) antigen, antibody to p24, and HIV-containing immune complexes in HIV-infected patients. J Infect Dis 158:1088

88. McSharry JJ, Pickering RJ, Caliguiri LA (1981) Activation of the alternate complement pathway by enveloped viruses containing limited amounts of sialic acid. Virology 114:507

89. Melchers F, Erdei A, Schultz T, Dierich MP (1985) Growth control of activated, synchronized murine B cells by the C3d fragment of human complement. Nature 317:264

90. Mizouchi T, Spellman MW, Larkin M, Solomon J, Basa LJ, Feizi T (1988) Carbohydrate structures of the human immunodeficiency virus (HIV) recombinant envelope glycoprotein gp120 produced in Chinese hamster ovary cells. Biochem J 254:599

91. Montefiori DC (1995) New insights into the role of host cell proteins in antiviral vaccine protection. AIDS Res Hum Retroviruses 11:1429

92. Montefiori DC (1996) Role of complement in HIV and SIV pathogenesis and immunity. In: Eible MM, Huber C, Peter HH, Wahn U (eds) Symposium in Immunology. V Antiviral Immunity. Springer, Heidelberg Berlin New York, pp 31–53

93. Montefiori DC, Robinson WE, Mitchell WM (1989) Antibody-independent, complement-mediated enhancement of HIV-1-infection by mannosidase I and II inhibitors. Antiviral Res 11:137

94. Montefiori DC, Robinson WE Jr, Hirsch VM, Modliszewski A, Mitchell WM, Johnson PR (1990) Antibody-dependent enhancement of simian immunodeficiency virus (SIV) infection in vitro by plasma from SIV-infected rhesus monkeys. J Virol 64:113

95. Montefiori DC, Lefkowitz LB, Keller RE, Holmberg V, Sandstrom E, Phair JP, the Multicenter AIDS Cohort Study Group (1991) Absence of a clinical correlation for complement-mediated, infection-enhancing antibodies in plasma and sera from HIV-1 infected persons. J Acquir Immune Defic Syndr 5:513

96. Montefiori DC, Graham BS, Kliks S, Wright PF, the NIAID AIDS Vaccine Clinical Trials Nework (1992) Serum antibodies to HIV-1 in recombinant vaccinia virus recipients boosted with purified recombinant gp160. J Clin Immunol 12:429

97. Montefiori DC, Zhou J, Shaff DI (1992) CD4-independent binding of HIV-1 to the B lymphocyte receptor CR2 (CD21) in the presence of complement and antibody. Clin Exp Immunol 90:383

98. Montefiori DC, Stewart K, Ahearn JM, Zhou JT, Zhou JY (1993) Complement-mediated binding of naturally glycosylated and glycosylation-modified human immunodeficiency virus type 1 to human CR2 (CD21). J Virol 67:2699

99. Montefiori DC, Cornell RJ, Zhou JY, Zhou JT, Hirsch VM, Johnson PR (1994) Complement control proteins, CD46, CD55, and CD59, as common surface constituents of human and simian immunodeficiency viruses and possible targets for vaccine protection. Virology 205:82

100. Montefiori DC, Graham BS, Zhou JY, Zhou JT, Ahearn JM (1994) Binding of human immunodeficiency virus type 1 to the C3b/C4b receptor, CR1 (CD35), and red blood cells in the presence of envelope-specific antibodies and complement. J Infect Dis 170:429

101. Montefiori DC, Reimann KA, Letvin NL, Zhou J, Hu S-L (1995) Studies of complement-activating antibodies in the SIV/macaque model of acute primary infection and vaccine protection. AIDS Res Hum Retroviruses 11:963

102. Montefiori DC, Pantaleo G, Fink LM, Zhou JT, Zhou JY, Bilska M, Miralles GD, Fauci AS (1996) Neutralizing and infection-enhancing antibody responses to human immunodeficiency virus type 1 in long-term nonprogressors. J Infect Dis 173:60

103. Morrow WJW, Wharton M, Stricker RB, Levy JA (1986) Circulating immune complexes in patients with acquired immune deficiency syndrome contain the AIDS-associated retrovirus. Clin Immunol Immunopathol 40:515
104. Muller-Eberhard H (1988) Molecular organization and function of the complement system. Annu Rev Biochem 57:321
105. Nikolova EB, Tomana M, Russell MW (1994) All forms of human IgA antibodies bound to antigen interfere with complement (C3) fixation induced by IgG or antigen alone. Scand J Immunol 39:275
106. Nikolova EB, Tomana M, Russell MW (1994) The role of the carbohydrate chains in complement (C3) fixation by solid-phase-bound human complement. Immunology 82:321
107. Nishanian P, Huskins KR, Stehn S, Detels R, Fahey JL (1990) A simple method for improved assay demonstrates that HIV p24 antigen is present as immune complexes in most sera from HIV-infected individuals. J Infect Dis 162:21
108. Pantaleo G, Fauci AS (1995) New concepts in the immunopathogenesis of HIV infection. Annu Rev Immunol 13:487
109. Pantaleo G, Graziosi C, Demarest JF, Cohen OJ, Vaccarezza, Gantt K, Muro-Cacho C, Fauci AS (1994) Role of lymphoid organs in the pathogenesis of human immunodeficiency virus (HIV) infection. Immunol Rev 140:105
110. Pardo V, Aldana M, Colton RM, Fischl MA, Jaffe D, Moskowitz L, Hensley GT, Burgoignie J (1984) Glomerular lesions in the acquired immunodeficiency syndrome. Ann Intern Med 101:429
111. Perelson AS, Neumann AU, Markowitz M, Leonard JM, Ho DD (1996) HIV-1 dynamics in vivo: virion clearance rate, infected cell life-span, and viral generation time. Science 271:1582
112. Perno C-F, Baseler MW, Broder S, Yarchoan R (1990) Infection of monocytes by human immunodeficiency virus type 1 blocked by inhibitors of CD4-gp120 binding, even in the presence of enhancing antibodies. J Exp Med 171:1043
113. Perricone R, Fontana L, De Carolis C, Carini C, Sirianni MC, Aiuti F (1987) Evidence for activation of complement in patients with AIDS related complex (ARC) and/or lymphadenopathy syndrome (LAS). Clin Exp Immunol 70:500
114. Pinter C, Siccardi AG, Longhi R, Clivio A (1995) Direct interaction of complement factor H with the C1 domain of HIV type 1 glycoprotein 120. AIDS Res Hum Retroviruses 11:577
115. Porterfield JS (1986) Antibody-dependent enhancement of viral infectivity. Adv Virus Res 31:335
116. Rademacher TW, Parekh RB, Dwek RA (1988) Glycobiology. Annu Rev Biochem 57:785
117. Ravetch JV, Kinet J-P (1991) Fc receptors. Annu Rev Immunol 9:457
118. Reisinger EC, Vogetseder W, Berzow D, Kofler D, Bitterlich G, Lehr HA, Wachter H, Dierich MP (1990) Complement-mediated enhancement of HIV-1-infection of the monoblastoid cell line U937. J Acquir Immune Defic Syndr 4:961
119. Reynes M, Aubert JP, Cohen JHM, Audouin J, Tricottet V, Diebold J, Kazatchkine MD (1985) Human follicular dendritic cells express CR1, CR2, and CR3 complement receptor antigens. J Immunol 135:2687
120. Robinson WE, Montefiori DC, Mitchell WM (1988) Antibody-dependent enhancement of human immunodeficiency virus type 1 infection. Lancet I:790
121. Robinson WE, Montefiori DC, Gillespie DH, Mitchell WM (1989) Complement-mediated, antibody-dependent enhancement of HIV-1-infection in vitro is characterized by increased protein and RNA synthesis and infectious virus release. J Acquir Immune Defic Syndr 2:33
122. Robinson WE, Kawamura T, Lake D, Masuho Y, Mitchell WM, Hersh EM (1990) Antibodies to the primary immunodominant domain of human immunodeficiency virus type 1 (HIV-1) glycoprotein gp41 enhance HIV-1-infection in vitro. J Virol 64:5301
123. Robinson WE, Montefiori DC, Mitchell WM (1990) Complement-mediated antibody-dependent enhancement of HIV-1 infection requires CD4 and complement receptors. Virology 175:600
124. Robinson WE, Gorny MW, Xu J-Y, Mitchell WM, Zolla-Pazner S (1991) Two immunodominant domains of gp41 bind antibodies which enhance human immunodeficiency virus type 1 infection in vitro. J Virol 65:4169
125. Ross GD, Medof E (1985) Membrane complement receptors specific for bound fragments of C3. Adv Immunol 37:217
126. Rosse WF (1987) The spleen as a filter. N Engl J Med 317:704
127. Rother RP, Rollins SA, Fodor WL, Albrecht J-C, Setter E, Fleckenstein B, Squinto SP (1994) Inhibition of complement-mediated cytolysis by the terminal complement inhibitor of herpesvirus saimiri. J Virol 68:730

128. Russell MW, Mansa B (1989) Complement-fixing properties of human IgA antibodies. Scand J Immunol 30:175

129. Saifuddin M, Parker CJ, Peeples ME, Gorny MK, Zolla-Pazner S, Ghassemi M, Rooney IA, Atkinson JP, Spear GT (1995) Role of virion-associated glycosylphosphatidylinositol-linked proteins CD55 and CD59 in complement resistance of cell line-derived and primary isolates of HIV-1. J Exp Med 182:501

130. Schifferli JA, Ng YC, Estreicher J, Walport MJ (1988) The clearance of tetanus toxoid-anti-tetanus toxoid immune complexes from the circulation of humans: complement- and erythrocyte CR1-dependent mechanisms. J Immunol 141:899

131. Schmitz J, Lunzen J van, Tenner-Racz K, Grosschupff G, Racz P, Schmitz H, Dietrich M, Hufert F (1994) Follicular dendritic cells (FDC) are not productively infected with HIV-1 in vivo. Adv Exp Med Biol 355:165

132. Schmitz J, Zimmer JP, Kluxen B, Aries S, Bogel M, Gigli I, Schmitz H (1995) Antibody-dependent complement-mediated cytotoxicity in sera from patients with HIV-1-infection is controlled by CD55 and CD59. J Clin Invest 95:1520

133. Schumaker V, Calcott M, Spiegelberg H, Muller-Eberhard H (1976) Ultracentrifuge studies of the binding of IgG of different subclasses to the C1q subunit of the first component of complement. Biochemistry 15:5175

134. Schupbach J, Tomasik Z, Jendis J, Boni J, Seger R, Kind C (1994) IgG, IgM, and IgA response to HIV in infants born to HIV-1 infected mothers. J AIDS 7:421

135. Scott, ME, Landay AL, Lint TF, Spear GT (1993) In vivo decrease in the expression of complement receptor 2 on B-cells in HIV infection. J Acquir Immune Defic Syndr 7:37

136. Senaldi G, Peakman M, McManus T, Davies ET, Tee DEH, Vergani D (1990) Activation of the complement system in human immunodeficiency virus infection: relevance of the classical pathway to pathogenesis and disease severity. J Infect Dis 162:1227

137. Senaldi G., Davies ET, Mahalingham M, Lu J, Pozniak A, Peakman M, Reid KBM, Vergani D (1995) Circulating levels of mannose binding protein in human immunodeficiency virus infection. J Infect 31:145

138. Serraino D, Salamina G, Franceschi S, Dubois D, La Vecchia C, Brunet JB, Ancelle-Park RA (1992) The epidemiology of AIDS-associated non-Hodgkin's lymphoma in the World Health Organization European Region. Br J Cancer 66:912

139. Shadduck PP, Weinberg JB, Haney AF, Bartlett JA, Langlois AJ, Bolognesi DP, Matthews TJ (1991) Lack of enhancing effect of human anti-human immunodeficiency virus type 1 (HIV-1) antibody on HIV-1-infection of human blood monocytes and peritoneal macrophages. J Virol 65:4309

140. Shirai A, Cosentino M, Leitman-Klinman SF, Klinman DM (1992) Human immunodeficiency virus infection induces both polyclonal and virus-specific B cell activation. J Clin Invest 89:561

141. Siebelink KHJ, Tijhaar E, Huisman RC, Huisman W, Ronde A de, Darby IH, Francis MJ, Rimmelzwaan GF, Osterhaus ADME (1995) Enhancement of feline immunodeficiency virus infection after immunization with envelope glycoprotein subunit vaccines. J Virol 69:3704

142. Smiley ML, Friedman HM (1985) Binding of complement component C3b to glycoprotein C is modulated by sialic acid on herpes simplex virus type 1-infected cells. J Virol 55:857

143. Soelder BM, Schultz TF, Hengster P, Lower J, Larcher C, Bitterlich G, Kurth R, Wachter H, Dierich MP (1989) HIV and HIV-infected cells differentially activate the human complement system independently of antibody. Immunol Lett 22:135

144. Soelder BM, Reisinger EC, Koefler D, Bitterlich G, Wachter H, Dierich MP (1989) Complement receptors: another port of entry for HIV. Lancet II:271

145. Spear GT, Jiang H, Sullivan BL, Gewurz H, Landay AL, Lint TF (1991) Direct binding of complement component C1q to human immunodeficiency virus (HIV) and human T lymphoptropic virus-I (HTLV-I) coinfected cells. AIDS Res Hum Retroviruses 7:579

146. Spear GT, Takefman DM, Sullivan BL, Landay AL, Jennings MB, Carlson JR (1993) Anti-cellular antibodies in sera from vaccinated macaques can induce complement-mediated virolysis of human immunodeficiency virus and simian immunodeficiency virus. Virology 195:475

147. Spiegelberg HL (1974) Biological activities of immunoglobulins of different classes and subclasses. Adv Immunol 19:259

148. Starcich BR, Hahn BH, Shaw GM, McNeely PD, Modrow S, Wolf H, Parks ES, Parks WP, Josephs SF, Gallo RC, Wong-Staal F (1986) Identification and characterization of conserved and variable regions in the envelope gene of HTLV-III/LAV, the retrovirus of AIDS. Cell 45:637

149. Stein BS, Gowda SD, Lifson JD, Penhallow RC, Bensch KG, Engleman EG (1987) pH-independent HIV entry into CD4-positive cells via virus envelope fusion to the plasma membrane. Cell 49:659
150. Stoiber H, Pinter C, Siccardi AG, Clivio, A, Dierich MP (1996) Efficient destruction of human immunodeficiency virus in human serum by inhibiting the protective action of complement factor H and decay accelerating factor (DAF, CD55). J Exp Med 183:307
151. Suga T, Endoh M, Sakai H, Miura M, Tomino Y, Nomoto Y (1985) T-alpha cell subsets in human peripheral blood. 1989. J Immunol 134:1327
152. Sundquist V-A, Linde A, Kurth R, Werner A, Helm EB, Popovic M, Gallo RC, Wahren B (1986) Restricted IgG subclass responses to HTLV-III/LAV and to cytomegalovirus in patients with AIDS and lymphadenopathy syndrome. J Infect Dis 153:970
153. Susal C, Kirschfink M, Kropelin M, Daniel V, Opelz G (1994) Complement activation by recombinant HIV-1 glycoprotein gp120. J Immunol 152:6028
154. Takeda A, Tuazon CU, Ennis FA (1988) Antibody-enhanced infection by HIV-1 via Fc receptor-mediated entry. Science 242:580
155. Takeda A, Sweet RW, Ennis FA (1990) Two receptors are required for antibody-dependent enhancement of human immunodeficiency virus type 1 infection: CD4 and FcγR. J Virol 64:5605
156. Tausk FA, McCutchan JA, Spechko P, Schreiber RD, Gigli I (1986) Altered erythrocyte C3b receptor expression, immune complexes, and complement activation in homosexual men in varying risk groups for acquired immune deficiency syndrome. J Clin Invest 78:977
157. Tedder TF, Clement LY, Cooper MD (1984) Expression of C3d receptors during human B cell differentiation: immunofluorescence analysis with the HB-5 monoclonal antibody. J Immunol 133:678
158. Tew JG, Mandel TE (1978) The maintenance and regulation of serum antibody levels: evidence indicating a role for antigen retained in lymphoid follicles. J Immunol 120:1063
159. Theil S (1992) Mannan-binding protein, a complement activating animal lectin. Immunopharmacology 24:91
160. Theiler M, Smith HH (1937) The use of yellow fever virus modified by in vitro cultivation for human immunization. J Exp Med 65:787
161. Thieblemont N, Haeffner-Cavaillon N, Ledur A, L'age-Stehr J, Ziegler-Heitbrock HWL, Kazatchkine MD (1993) CR1 (CD35) and CR3 (CD11b/CD18) mediate infection of human monocytes and monocytic cell lines with complement-opsonized HIV independently of CD4. Clin Exp Immunol 92:106
162. Thieblemont N, Haeffner-Cavaillon N, Weiss L, Maillet F, Kazatchkine MD (1993) Complement activation by gp160 glycoprotein of HIV-1. AIDS Res Hum Retroviruses 9:229
163. Thielens NM, Bally IM, Ebenbichler CF, Dierich, MP, Arlaud GJ (1993) Further characterization of the interaction between the C1q subcomponent of human C1 and the transmembrane envelope glycoprotein gp41 of HIV-1. J Immunol 151:6583
164. Thyphronitis G, Kinoshita T, Inoue K, Schweinle JE, Tsokos GC, Mecalf ES, Finkelman FD, Balow JE (1991) Modulation of mouse complement receptors 1 and 2 suppresses antibody response in vivo. J Immunol 147:224
165. Toth FD, Mosborg-Petersen P, Kiss J, Aboagye-Mathiesen G, Zdravkovic M, Hager H, Aranyosi J, Lampe L, Ebbesen P (1994) Antibody-dependent enhancement of HIV-1-infection in human term syncytiotrophoblast cells cultured in vitro. Clin Exp Immunol 96:389
166. Tremblay M, Meloche S, Sekaly RP, Wainberg MA (1990) Complement receptor type 2 mediates enhancement of human immunodeficiency virus type 1 infection in Epstein-Barr virus-carrying B cells. J Exp Med 171:1791
167. Trischmann H, Davis D, Lachmann PJ (1995) Lymphocytic strains of HIV-1 when complexed with enhancing antibodies can infect macrophages via FcγRIII, independently of CD4. AIDS Res Hum Retroviruses 11:343
168. Tsokos GC, Lambris JD, Finkelman FD, Anastassiou ED, June CH (1990) Monovalent ligands of complement receptor 2 inhibit, whereas polyvalent ligands enhance anti-Ig-induced human B cell intracytoplasmic-free calcium concentration. J Immunol 144:1640
169. Veronese FM, DeVico AL, Copeland TD, Droszland S, Gallo RC, Sarngadharan MG (1985) Characterization of gp41 as the transmembrane protein coded by the HTLV-III/LAV envelope gene. Science 229:1402
170. Wang S Z-S, Rushlow KE, Issel CJ, Cook RF, Cook SJ, Raabe ML, Chong Y-H, Costa L, Montelaro RC (1994) Enhancement of EIAV replication and disease by immunization with a baculovirus-expressed recombinant envelope surface glycoprotein. Virology 199:247

171. Wei X, Ghosh SK, Taylor ME, Johnson VA, Emini EA, Deutsch P, Lifson, JD, Bonhoeffer S, Nowak MA, Hahn BH, Saag MS, Shaw GM (1995) Viral dynamics in human immunodeficiency virus type 1 infection. Nature 373:117

172. Weiss L, Okada N, Haeffner-Cavaillon N, Hattori C, Faucher C, Kazatchkine MD, Okada H (1992) Decreased expression of the membrane inhibitor of complement-mediated cytolysis CD59 on T-lymphocytes of HIV-infected patients. J Acquir Immune Defic Syndr 6:379

173. Wilson BS, Platt JL, Kay NE (1985) Monoclonal antibodies to the 140,000 mol wt glycoprotein of B lymphocyte membranes (CR2 receptor) initiates proliferation of B cells in vitro. Blood 66:824

174. Wu XS, Okada N, Iwamori M, Okada H (1996) IgM natural antibody against an asialo-oligosaccharide, gangliotetraose (GG4), sensitizes HIV-1-infected cells for cytolysis by homologous complement. Int Immunol 8:153

175. Yefenof E, Asjo B, Klein E (1991) Alternative complement pathway activation by HIV infected cells: C3 fixation does not lead to complement lysis but enhances NK sensitivity. Int Immunol 3:395

176. Zeira M, Byrn RA, Groopman JE (1990) Inhibition of serum-enhanced HIV-1-infection of U937 monocytoid cells by recombinant soluble CD4 and anti-CD4 monoclonal antibody. AIDS Res Hum Retroviruses 6:629

Simian immunodeficiency virus as a model of HIV pathogenesis

Stephen Norley, Reinhard Kurth

Paul-Ehrlich-Institute, Paul-Ehrlich-Strasse 51–59, D-63225 Langen, Germany

Introduction

HIV and AIDS have been an ever increasingly important component of the health risks facing Man worldwide for more than a decade. The potential for a massive and crippling epidemic has prompted intense efforts to develop vaccines and anti-viral therapeutics. However, despite great advances, particularly over the last few years, in our understanding of how the virus interacts with its host and of how to treat the infection, the fundamental reasons for the breakdown of the immune system which leads to the development of AIDS are still not known. Determining how HIV causes AIDS would enormously help the development of treatments for patients whose immune systems are eroded by HIV infection.

The simian immunodeficiency virus (SIV) model for HIV pathogenesis is being increasingly used to help solve the riddle of AIDS; but why use an animal model at all when there are millions of humans infected with HIV itself? After all, a model, no matter how useful, is only a model and the lessons learned might not relate to human AIDS. In answer to this question we will, in this review, point out the striking similarities between simian AIDS induced by SIV and the disease induced in humans by AIDS. In addition the opportunities that the SIV/monkey model offer for studying the virus-host relationship under precisely defined conditions will be described.

Origins and characteristics of SIV

In the last 10 years a multitude of SIV strains have been isolated from a variety of monkey (and ape) species. These have been characterized both in vitro and in vivo and for the most part sequenced molecular clones are available. For most isolates, no evidence for infection of the relevant monkey species can be found in the wild – most infections occur in primate colonies only. The most important exceptions are sooty

---

Correspondence to: S. Norley

mangabeys and African green monkeys, a large percentage of which are naturally infected with SIV_{sm} and SIV_{agm}, respectively [42, 59], and which, as described later, do not succumb to AIDS. Moreover, most of the 'unnatural' AIDS-inducing infections in primate colonies appear to have resulted from the accidental transmission of SIV_{sm} into heterologous species. SIV_{mac} (rhesus macaques), SIV_{mne} (pig-tailed macaques), SIV_{cyn} (cynomolgus macaques) and others all share a close genetic relationship with SIV_{sm} [55]. Indeed, HIV-2, more prevalent in Africa than in the Western world, is a close relation of SIV_{sm} which almost certainly represents the source of this zoonosis [36].

Most of the HIV-related studies in lower primates has been performed using rhesus or cynomolgus macaques infected with SIV_{mac}. SIV_{mac} is a lentivirus which has not only a close genetic relationship to HIV-1 (and even more so to HIV-2) but also interacts with its host cell in a remarkably similar fashion. In fact, the use in recent years of primary HIV-1 isolates has shown that SIV_{mac} is, in many ways, more reminiscent of 'real' HIV-1 than are the T cell-adapted laboratory strains used in most of the initial studies of HIV-1.

The SIV model is predominantly an invaluable tool for the initial development and testing of vaccines [65]. Groups of immunized animals can be challenged with a known dose of a cloned and sequenced virus at the time of peak immune response, allowing vaccine efficacy to be determined using a relatively low number of subjects. However, the availability of different SIV isolates and clones has also made the study of AIDS pathogenesis at the molecular level possible. Isolates and clones of SIV are now available which range in their pathogenicity, depending on the monkey species, from apathogenic (no disease induction) to acutely pathogenic (death within 6 days). Not only can the pathogenic potential of identical viruses in different host species be studied, but also the effect of deleting or exchanging individual viral genes or gene fragments. These properties have made SIV an invaluable tool for studying the events leading to the development of AIDS.

Apathogenic SIV infection of the natural host

At first, studying an apathogenic infection in the hope of learning something about the pathogenesis of AIDS might seem counter-intuitive. However, the interaction between HIV-1 and the host is highly complex, making it almost impossible to discern the primary mechanism(s) of disease induction. By comparing the virus-host interactions in pathogenic and apathogenic infections, however, it should be possible at least to eliminate putative disease mechanisms. The two SIV/natural host systems studied most intensely have been SIV_{sm} infection of sooty mangabeys and SIV_{agm} infection of African green monkeys (AGMs).

As mentioned above, mangabeys infected for most of their lives in the wild with SIV_{sm} show no signs of developing immunodeficiency disease. The virus itself clearly has the potential for pathogenicity in the correct setting as accidental or experimental transfer of the virus to heterologous species of monkeys has resulted in the emergence of a wide spectrum of isolates able to induce AIDS. In fact, the diversity of the HIV-2 epidemic in certain regions of Africa is almost certainly the result of SIV_{sm} entering the human population by independent cross-species events [36]. The differences between infection of the natural versus heterologous host are not simply the result of selection for pathogenic strains by serial passage through a different species: inoculation of the same virus into monkeys will result in an almost inapparent infection in the case of sooty mangabeys and the rapid development of AIDS in the case of the heterologous host [69]. Clearly, the host plays an important role in determining the outcome of the infection.

Although, like SIV_{sm}, SIV_{agm} infects a large proportion of its natural host species without causing disease, transfer of the virus to different monkey species initially failed to result in AIDS [34]. Unlike SIV_{sm}, it therefore seemed possible that SIV_{agm} is simply apathogenic per se, lacking the properties needed for disease induction. Recently, however, Hirsch et al. [38] have generated by serial passage an isolate and molecular clone of SIV_{agm} able to cause the rapid onset of disease in pig-tailed macaques. SIV_{agm}, therefore, also has a deadly potential in the right setting.

Virus load and variability

The most obvious possibility to explain the lack of disease in the natural sooty mangabey and AGM hosts would be a failure of the virus to grow efficiently. However, there is no evidence that the in vivo virus load of SIV_{agm} or SIV_{sm} in their respective hosts is any lower than that seen during pathogenic SIV or HIV infections, at least during the asymptomatic phase. Indeed, sooty mangabeys appear to have, if anything, a relatively high amount of virus in circulation [31]. The number of infected cells in the blood of AGMs as measured by limiting co-culture analysis or polymerase chain reaction (PCR) is similar to that seen in HIV-1-infected asymptomatic humans, although it never appears to rise to the levels often associated with disease progression [35]. It is also possible to isolate live virus from the plasma of infected AGMs, showing that the animals are subjected to an active, ongoing infection. Indeed, recent data suggest that the levels of virus, as measured by RNA copies in circulation, might even be higher than that seen during HIV-infection (P. Johnson, personal communication).

One of the outstanding features of HIV-1 is its capacity for rapid genomic change, predominantly the consequence of errors made by reverse transcriptase. The degree of variation within both the population and the individual is very high, hindering attempts to develop effective vaccines and therapeutic agents. It has long been thought possible that HIV persists by continually escaping from immune control, leading eventually to exhaustion and breakdown of the immune system. The fidelity of the SIV_{agm} reverse transcriptase, however, is similar to that of HIV-1 [52] and when isolates from different animals are compared, a high degree of genomic variation is obvious [3]. Inoculation of AGMs with a molecular clone of SIV_{agm} and subsequent sequence analysis reveals a degree of in vivo variability similar to that observed for HIV-1 in humans [4].

Antiviral immune response and soluble factors

As one might expect given the comparable in vivo virus burden, the antiviral immune response in infected mangabeys and AGMs does not appear to be particularly more effective than in the pathogenic systems. AGMs, for example, develop antibodies able to bind viral proteins and antibodies initiating antibody-dependent cellular cytolysis (ADCC) of infected cells [56], similar to HIV-1-infected humans. Also similar to that seen in humans are the low levels of neutralizing antibody and weak or absent complement-mediated cytolysis response. One interesting difference is the weak or absent humoral immune response to the viral Gag protein [56], despite high levels of antibodies reacting to other (e.g., Env) proteins. Inoculation of a cloned virus into naive AGMs results in little or no anti-Gag antibodies, whereas a strong anti-Gag response is seen with the same virus in heterologous species. Whether this failure to react to Gag plays a role in the animals' resistance to disease is as yet unknown, and will be discussed later, but it is perhaps significant that some sooty mangabeys infected with SIV_{sm} also fail to mount a humoral immune response to this protein [31]. Cytotoxic T lymphocytes (CTL) are considered to be the major immune mechanism against viral infection and HIV-1-infected humans have an extraordinarily high level of circulating CTL precursors specific for the virus [14]. Possibly due to a number of technical difficulties, it has not yet been possible to reproducibly demonstrate virus-specific CTLs in SIV_{agm}-infected AGMs. However, even in the SIV_{sm}/sooty mangabey system, in which the necessary tools and reagents are available and have been shown to work in heterologous hosts, CTLs have been very elusive [32]. Again, this lack of a particular immune response in a natural, apathogenic virus/host may tell us a lot about the mechanisms of pathogenesis.

There has been, for some years now, a great deal of effort directed at identifying the soluble factor(s) secreted by $CD8^+$ lymphocytes which has the capability to suppress HIV replication in vitro. The existence of the factor(s), or at least the effect, has been demonstrated in virtually all SIV systems tested [24, 43]. Although the in vivo role in controlling virus replication remains unknown, it might be significant that AGMs (in whose cells the factor has been demonstrated [26]) have a relatively high proportion of $CD8^+$ cells in circulation [26]. Recently, a number of molecules have been identified which appear to be at least partially responsible for the suppressive effect of $CD8^+$ cells. The chemokines MIP-1α, MIP-1β and RANTES [18] and the interleukin (IL)-16 molecule [5] are all secreted by $CD8^+$ cells and can suppress virus replication. Moreover, the cellular receptors for the chemokines have been shown to act as co-receptors for virus entry [21].

Virus trapping in lymph nodes

As will be discussed later, it has been demonstrated in recent years that a disproportionately high burden of virus exists in the lymph nodes of HIV-infected humans, even during the asymptomatic phase of the infection [60]. Most of this virus appears to be trapped at the surface of dendritic cells rather than being actively produced in the nodes [25, 64]. Perhaps as a result of this trapping or by some other mechanism, the lymph nodes of infected patients are systematically destroyed as disease progresses, so that eventually little of the fine structure (and presumably functionality) remains. If one looks at the lymph nodes of AGMs during SIV_{agm} infection, they too show active virus replication during the initial few weeks which then disappears, similar to the nodes of SIV_{mac}-infected macaques. However, unlike humans and macaques, no accumulation of trapped virus occurs in the ensuing months or years with the overall virus burden remaining similar to that seen in the blood [11]. It is not surprising, therefore, that the fine architecture of AGM lymph nodes, even after many years of ongoing SIV_{agm} infection, remains intact.

Pathogenic infection of the heterologous host

As mentioned above, the clinical outcome of SIV infection depends upon both the isolate or molecular clone and the monkey species used. The majority of studies have been carried out using one of the SIV_{mac} or SIV_{sm} isolates which induce a disease pattern very similar to that of human AIDS, albeit in a compressed time frame. Following intravenous, intrarectal or intravaginal infection, animals develop fever and often a erythematous maculopapular skin rash containing a massive infiltration of $CD8^+$ lymphocytes, which parallels the development of plasma viremia (after 1–2 weeks). This rise in viremia is also associated with a transient drop in the number of circulating $CD4^+$ cells. In the majority of animals, as the antiviral immune response becomes evident (CTLs as early as 6 days after infection and neutralizing antibodies at 2–3 weeks), the circulating viral antigen is rapidly cleared and the $CD4^+$ cell numbers return to near normal. Infected monkeys then enter a period in which clinical signs of infection are negligible apart from the presence of lymphadenopathy. However, this asymptomatic phase almost certainly hides an ongoing titanic struggle between the virus and the immune system, similar to that recently revealed in HIV-infected humans, with the whole body burden of virus and virus-infected cells being eliminated and replenished every few days [39, 70]. During this time, which for SIV infection is usually 3 months to 3 years, the circulating $CD4^+$ cell count gradually declines. Eventually, however, infected monkeys will experience a drop in antiviral antibodies, a rise in viremia, a calamitous drop in $CD4^+$ cells and body weight and the development of persistent diarrhoea. Such full-blown simian AIDS lasts only a few weeks or months before it is necessary to euthanize the animal.

The sequence of events at the macroscopic and cellular level following infection and during progression to disease is now slowly becoming clearer. Although most studies have understandably concentrated on the patterns of infection in the blood, it appears that the major sites of infection and damage are the various lymphoid tissues and bone marrow. For example, as early as 3 days postinoculation it is possible to detect SIV-infected monocyte/macrophages in the bone marrow. Moreover, the acute phase of infection is associated with macrophage, myeloid and megakaryocytic hyperplasia, and macrophage activation in the bone marrow [51]. Similarly, SIV-infected cells appear in the gut-associated lymphoid tissue within 7 days of infection, before blood-associated infection becomes apparent (J. Stott, personal communication). Lackner et al. [46] found the major sites of infection at 2 weeks postinfection to be the thymus and spleen, and Persidsky et al. [61] identified virus-containing Kupffer cells present in the majority of livers tested as early as 4 days postinoculation. Whatever the primary site(s) of infection, SIV rapidly disseminates to the majority of lymphoid organs; indeed autopsy of animals with AIDS reveals the virus disseminated throughout the body, with SIV proviral DNA present in nearly all lymphoid and non-lymphoid tissues [37].

Persistent SIV infection has a catastrophic effect on the fine structure of the lymphoid organs, in particular the thymus and lymph nodes. Thymic atrophy and a profound reduction of thymic lymphocyte numbers is common in macaques with AIDS [9]. In situ hybridization of lymph nodes reveals massive viral replication during the first week of infection after which time infected cells virtually disappear and viral RNA is found predominantly in the germinal centers in the form of virus trapped by follicular dendritic cells [16, 40]. Thereafter, follicular hyperplasia and depletion can occur with total disruption of the lymph node fine structure as AIDS progresses.

HIV effects not only the cells of the immune system but is also increasingly associated with lesions in the nervous system [66]. A similar neural pathology is often observed during SIV infection of macaques [8, 45, 68], with a perivascular accumulation of macrophages in the brain and spinal cord. Infection of the central nervous system (CNS) is an early event, with SIV detectable as early as 7 days after inoculation [15] and the viruses responsible for CNS infection appear to be especially adapted genetically for that environment [47].

As with HIV-1-infection of humans, the progressive breakdown of the immune system in SIV-infected monkeys is associated with the development of opportunistic infections. The nature of the diseases associated with simian AIDS will obviously depend on the microorganisms prevalent in the monkey colony. Viral, bacterial, fungal and protozoal infections can all lead to opportunistic disease, many of which are commonly seen with human AIDS. For example, cytomegalovirus (CMV) infections are common in both human and simian AIDS, with SIV-infected macaques often showing evidence of CMV in a wide variety of organs [7]. Pneumonia due to *Pneumoscystis carinii* infection is often observed in infected monkeys [67] and *Candida* infections of the oral cavity or esophagus have been documented. *Mycobacterium avium* complex (MAC) in macaques closely resembles the disease commonly associated with HIV infection of humans, with the spleen, liver, gastrointestinal tract and lymph nodes most often involved [67]. Interestingly, a recent study [53] showed that the strain of SIV used to infect the macaque influences the likelihood of MAC development and that MAC is associated with *prolonged* survival after primary infection.

It is, therefore, clear that the range of symptoms and diseases resulting from SIV infection of macaques is strikingly similar to that associated with human AIDS. This allows novel therapeutic approaches to be initially evaluated in the SIV-infected macaque before human trials are performed. There are, as with any model, differences between human and simian AIDS, particularly in the period of time between infection and disease development. Also, Kaposi's sarcoma, so often observed with HIV-infected humans, does not commonly develop during SIV-associated simian AIDS. However, the similarities far outweigh the differences and SIV infection of macaques will continue to be a valuable tool in the study of AIDS.

Acutely pathogenic SIV

The strains of SIV described in the section above all cause the development of disease similar to human AIDS and studying how the pathogenicity of SIV is influenced by passage through different monkey species has been enormously informative. The potential for phenotypic change is, however, best exemplified by PBj14, a variant of SIV_{sm} able to induce an acute form of disease in macaques, resulting in death within 1 or 2 weeks of infection [30]. PBj14, in the forms of an isolate or, biological or molecular clones causes the rapid onset of fulminant diarrhoea and acidosis in pig-tailed macaques [48], with infected animals showing a high level of virus in circulation and in the gut-associated lymphoid tissue. Animals surviving the initial acute phase of the disease enter a 'normal' asymptomatic phase of infection and eventually develop simian AIDS, similar to the course of infection with the parental strain. The acute form of disease is never observed with HIV infection of humans (or SIV_{mac} infection of macaques) and its relevance to AIDS is debatable. Some laboratories, however, have used the model in vaccine trials to avoid the 3- to 36-month waiting period required when the end-point of the vaccine trial is disease development.

PBj14 has taught us some valuable lessons concerning the way in which the virus interacts with the host, and the acute disease that it causes may represent an extreme example of what is happening during infection with 'normal' SIV. In vitro, PBj14 has the unusual feature of being able to grow well in unstimulated peripheral blood mononuclear cells (PBMCs) [29], unlike HIV-1 and other SIV strains which require cells to be exogenously stimulated (for example by a mitogen) for efficient replication to occur. PBj14 does not require addition of mitogens because it appears to have the ability to stimulate the cells itself.

Monkeys infected with PBj14 suffer an extreme overexpression of the cytokine IL-6 [12], and it is almost certainly cytokine dysfunction which results in the symptoms of the acute disease. Induction of cytokine expression and stimulation of PBMCs is reminiscent of the effects of superantigens on lymphocytes and indeed, PBj14 has been shown to stimulate expansion of Vβ7- and Vβ14-expressing T lymphocytes both in vitro and in vivo [17].

The production of closely related, sequenced molecular clones of SIV, one of which causes acute disease and others which do not, obviously provides a means of identifying the genetic determinants of disease induction. A number of studies have been performed using chimeric viruses carrying different gene fragments of PBj14 [20, 58], but the most elegant and informative studies have been recently published by Du et al. [22], who showed that substituting just two amino acids in the Nef protein of SIV$_{mac}$239 converted the virus from a 'normal' AIDS-inducing clone to one causing acute, PBj14-like disease. Further studies showed that even a single amino acid change at position 17 of Nef from arginine to tyrosine confers the acute phenotype and, conversely, changing the tyrosine to arginine at the same position in PBj14 abrogated this property [23]. Although other studies [20] show that the genetic background in which the PBj14 nef gene is expressed is crucial, these studies clearly demonstrate the importance of Nef in the acute pathogenesis of PBj14. The results are also consistent with the emerging view of nef function in SIV and HIV which result from studies using nef deletion mutants (discussed in the next section).

Deletion mutants and hybrid viruses

As stated in the introduction, one of the most obvious advantages of the SIV animal model for AIDS is that it allows the genetic determinants of pathogenesis to be studied. Such studies usually take one of two forms: either a gene is deleted and the function of the gene is then inferred by observing the phenotypic changes that occur or genes are exchanged between pathogenic and apathogenic clones of SIV. Studies of this nature obviously cannot be performed in the HIV/human system and as the effects of genetic manipulation are often quite different in vivo compared with in vitro, the SIV model has been invaluable in determining immunodeficiency virus gene function.

Desrosiers and colleagues [44] first showed that, whereas deletion of the nef gene had little effect on the ability of SIV$_{mac}$ to grow in tissue culture, such deletion mutants were severely compromised in their replicative capacity in vivo. The in vivo viral load achieved by SIV$_{mac}\Delta$nef is dramatically reduced compared to its full length parental strain and it quickly becomes difficult to isolate the virus, with animals remaining healthy with no signs of disease progression for many years. Removal of the additional genes vpr and NRE to create $SIV_{mac}\Delta 3$ resulted in a virus with an even more extremely attenuated phenotype, although infection and seroconversion were readily demonstrated [72]. In addition to the providing evidence for the importance of Nef in vivo, the attenuated virus mutants have been predominantly used within the framework of vaccine studies. Animals infected with nef deletion mutants of SIV_{mac} are often totally resistant to subsequent infection with the pathogenic wild-type virus [1, 19, 57]. Although it is unlikely, due to understandable safety concerns, that a live attenuated form of HIV-1 would be used as an AIDS vaccine in the general population in the foreseeable future, the protection afforded by this form of virus in the SIV system is orders of magnitude better than that achieved with other forms of vaccine. Identifying the mechanism(s) of protection has therefore been, and remains, a high priority goal in the hope that a similar state of immunity can be stimulated using a less hazardous form of vaccine.

In contrast to its highly attenuated phenotype in adult macaques, the $SIV_{mac}\Delta 3$ deletion mutant has been shown to cause the rapid onset of simian AIDS in newborn animals [2]. This result, as well as reducing further the chances for using live attenuated viruses in humans, provides further information about the in vivo role of Nef. The notion that newborn animals are so highly susceptible to AIDS induction that even an attenuated virus can cause disease is probably wrong. It is more likely that Nef is redundant in newborn macaques, as it is in cell culture. Indeed, full-length but attenuated clones of SIV induce no more disease in neonates than they do in adults [54].

The importance of Nef in AIDS pathogenesis was nicely demonstrated recently in an experiment which nature performed for us. Rhesus macaques were infected with the $SIV_{mac}32H$ C8 molecular clone, whose major difference from the full-length pathogenic J5 clone is a four amino acid deletion in the Nef protein [62]. Most animals, as expected, experienced a course of infection typical for the attenuated clones described above. In one animal, however, the virus mutated to fill in the deletion by a repeat of flanking sequences and then proceeded to alter the amino acids one at a time until the original, full-length sequence was restored [71]. Consequently, the virus burden in this animal increased dramatically and AIDS soon followed.

There has been a lot of interest in the past few years in the development of SIV/HIV hybrids, or 'SHIVs'. These viruses offer the possibility of testing, for example, a candidate AIDS vaccine based on the HIV-1 envelope glycoprotein in lower primates. Animals could be immunized with the vaccine and the immune responses analyzed and, if appropriate, the monkeys could be challenged with a SHIV in which the SIV envelope gene has been replaced with that of HIV-1. SHIVs are also a useful tool for analyzing gene function in vivo. Genes from HIV-1 clones showing particular in vitro characteristics can be expressed in a SHIV and the in vivo characteristics examined. In one study, a SHIV carrying the tat, rev and env genes of a T cell tropic, syncitia-forming HIV-1 molecular clone was shown to replicate in macaques with an efficiency orders of magnitude higher that a SHIV carrying the same genes from a macrophage-tropic, non-syncitium-forming clone [50]. Initially even SHIVs based on the pathogenic $SIV_{mac}239$ clone failed to induce disease in macaques, and it seemed that the exchange of genes had effectively attenuated the virus [49, 63]. Recently, however, serial passage of one such 'attenuated' SHIV in pig-tailed macaques succeeded in producing an isolate causing progressive loss of $CD4^+$ cells and development of AIDS [41]. As well as offering an improved model for vaccine evaluation, it will be of great interest to determine which of the relatively few genomic changes that occurred during the passage are responsible for converting an apathogenic virus to a pathogenic SHIV.

Mechanisms of pathogenesis

Despite the overwhelming amount of data accumulated during the study of human and simian AIDS the precise biological events which result in the progression to disease remain unknown. Although HIV and SIV predominantly infect the cells of the immune system, there are simply not enough infected cells in the blood (or lymph nodes) of the infected individual to account for the dramatic collapse of immunity. The milestone work by Ho et al. [39] and Wei et al. [70] showing that the entire population of virus and actively infected cells in the body are eliminated and replaced every few days has led to speculation about 'immune exhaustion' as a reason for immune dysfunction. Even so, the apparent excess of uninfected CD4+ cells in the body has prompted researchers to look for indirect mechanisms of immune cell depletion.

One of the more popular proposals suggests that CD4+ cells are eliminated by inappropriate induction of programmed cell death (apoptosis). A sizeable proportion of lymphocytes from HIV-1-infected humans have been shown to be primed for apoptosis and when stimulated ex vivo these cells self-destruct instead of proliferating [33]. In addition cross-linking of the CD4 molecule by HIV-1 envelope glycoprotein and gp120-specific antibody has been shown to prime cells for apoptosis [6], and apoptotic cells can be readily demonstrated in the disrupted thymi of HIV-1-infected patients [13]. The question of whether programmed cell death is the cause or merely the result of immune dysfunction during AIDS is a difficult one to answer. It is perhaps significant, however, that apoptosis of CD4+ cells could be readily shown [27] in those systems resulting in disease (HIV-1 in humans, SIV_{mac} in rhesus macaques) but not in those in which no disease occurs (nonpathogenic SIV_{mac} clone in rhesus, HIV-1 in chimpanzees, SIV_{agm} in AGMs).

As described earlier, the acute disease resulting from infection with the unusual PBj14 variant of SIV_{sm} is almost certainly the result of massive overproduction of cytokines, and this phenotype appears to be due to minor changes in the nef gene. The Nef protein of the 'normal' immunodeficiency viruses shares some of these properties, albeit at a reduced level, and inappropriate expression of IL-6 and tumor necrosis factor (TNF)-α has been demonstrated in the lymph nodes of people with both early and late stage disease [28]. It therefore seems possible that unrelenting disturbance of the cytokine network by HIV or SIV, perhaps as a result of a superantigen-like effect, could lead to or contribute to the erosion of the immune system.

The massive accumulation of virus in the lymph nodes of HIV-1-infected humans and SIV-infected macaques [10, 64] and eventual disturbance and destruction of lymph node architecture and function is likely to be one of the most important causes of immunodeficiency disease. After all, it is within the fine structure of the lymph nodes that the cellular interactions and signaling needed for initiation of the immune response to a pathogen occur. As mentioned earlier, the lymph nodes are destroyed in the absence of massive infection and it would appear that an indirect mechanism must be responsible. Certainly, inappropriate apoptosis is one candidate for this role, but the extensive trapping of virus and, presumably, immune complexes within the nodes suggests that immunopathological mechanisms (i.e., destruction of uninfected cells by immune mechanisms directed at the trapped virus) might also play an important role in the demise of the lymph node. In this regard it is tempting to suggest the following (highly speculative) model to account for the apathogenicity of SIV_{agm} and SIV_{sm} in their natural hosts (Fig. 1). As mentioned earlier, SIV_{agm}-infected AGM develop no (or low levels of) antibodies specific for Gag and this would preclude the formation of immune complexes containing immature virus particles perhaps released by the action of CTLs. This in turn might account for the failure of SIV_{agm} to accumulate detrimentally in the lymph nodes, with the virus particles remaining instead in circulation. There are naturally problems with the model: for example the inability so far to demonstrate SIV_{agm}-specific CTLs and the lack of evidence for anti-gag antibody/virus particle immune complexes during pathogenic HIV and SIV infection. However, the model fits the observations of low anti-gag antibody, high circulating virus and lack of trapped virus in the lymph nodes during apathogenic SIV_{agm} infection of its natural host. Hopefully, ongoing investigations will soon validate or disprove the hypothesis.

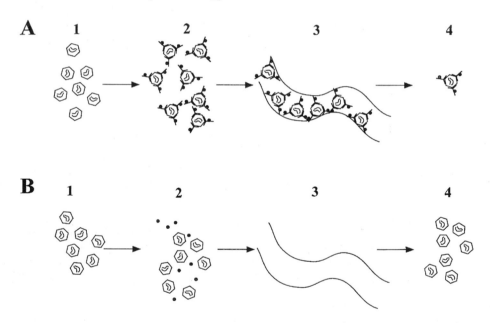

Fig. 1A, B. Hypothetical model of how a lack of anti-Gag antibodies during simian immunodeficiency virus (SIV)$_{agm}$ infection might account for lack of virus trapping in the lymph nodes. During pathogenic HIV or SIV infection (**A**), immature non-infectious virus particles, possibly released as a result of cytotoxic T lymphocyte-mediated cell lysis (*1*), are rapidly coated (*2*) by anti-Gag antibodies and complement (•). These complexes become trapped (*3*) in the lymph nodes by Fc or C′ receptors, reducing the viral load in circulation (*4*). Lymph node cells coated in immune complexes (as shown by in situ hybridization or immunostaining) become susceptible to immunopathological attack, resulting in the eventual destruction of the lymph node architecture. In contrast (**B**) immature particles (*1*) released during SIV_{agm} infection are not coated by antibody (*2*) and so pass through the lymph nodes (*3*) to return to the circulation (*4*)

Conclusions

In conclusion, it is obvious that the study of the various SIV/primate systems available have contributed significantly to our understanding of how an immunodeficiency virus interacts with its host. This has come partially from the comparison of pathogenic versus nonpathogenic systems and partially from studies in which genes are deleted or exchanged. The disease induced by the pathogenic strains (or clones) of SIV_{mac} is remarkably similar to human AIDS, although developing within a conveniently shorter period of time. The ability to dissect events at the physiological, cellular and genetic levels during infection and progression to disease has been a valuable tool in this field. In addition, studying the biological interactions occurring during the almost inapparent infection of the natural host and the devastating illness induced by the aberrant PBj14 strain has given many insights into the possible causes of immune dysfunction.

There are, however, still large gaps in our understanding of precisely how and why HIV and SIV infection results ultimately in AIDS. Hopefully, with the new technologies becoming available the combination of knowledge gleaned from the studies of HIV in humans and SIV in primates will allow these gaps to be filled in the near future.

Table 1. Comparison of pathogenic and nonpathogenic systems

	Pathogenic systems (HIV/humans, SIV_{mac}/macaque)	Nonpathogenic system SIV_{agm}/AGM
Peripheral viral load	Moderately high during asymptomatic phase, increasing with disease progression	Equally high (or even higher)
In vivo variability	High	High
Humoral immune response	Strong	Strong (low or absent response to Gag)
Cellular immune response	Strong	Not yet reproducibly demonstrated
Lymph nodes	Trapping of virus at the surface of cells; eventual destruction of lymph node architecture	No trapping of virus in lymph nodes; architecture remains intact
Priming of CD4$^+$ cells for apoptosis	Yes	No

SIV, Simian immunodeficiency virus; AGM, African green monkey

References

1. Almond N, Kent K, Cranage M, Rud E, Clarke B, Stott EJ (1995) Protection by attenuated simian immunodeficiency virus in macaques against challenge with virus-infected cells. Lancet 345:1342
2. Baba TW, Jeong YS, Penninck D, Bronson R, Greene MF, Ruprecht RM (1995) Pathogenicity of live attenuated SIV after mucosal infection of neonatal macaques. Science 267:1820
3. Baier M, Werner A, Cichutek K, Garber C, Mueller C, Kraus G, Ferdinand FJ, Hartung S, Papas TS, Kurth R (1989) Molecularly cloned simian immunodeficiency virus SIVagm3 is highly divergent from other SIVagm isolates and is biologically active in vitro and in vivo. J Virol 63:5119
4. Baier M, Dittmar MT, Cichutek K, Kurth R (1991) Development in vivo of genetic variability of simian immunodeficiency virus. Proc Natl Acad Sci USA 88:8126
5. Baier M, Werner A, Bannert N, Metzner K, Kurth R (1995) HIV suppression by interleukin-16. Nature 378:563

6. Banda NK, Bernier J, Kurahara DK, Kurrle R, Haigwood N, Sekaly RP, Finkel TH (1992) Crosslinking CD4 by human immunodeficiency virus gp120 primes T cells for activation-induced apoptosis. J Exp Med 176:1099
7. Baskin GB (1987) Disseminated cytomegalovirus infection in immunodeficient rhesus monkeys. Am J Pathol 129:345
8. Baskin GB, Murphey-Corb M, Watson EA, Martin LN (1988) Necropsy findings in rhesus monkeys experimentally infected with cultured simian immunodeficiency virus (SIV)/delta. Vet Pathol 25:456
9. Baskin GB, Murphey CM, Martin LN, Davison FB, Hu FS, Kuebler D (1991) Thymus in simian immunodeficiency virus-infected rhesus monkeys. Lab Invest 65:400
10. Baskin GB, Martin LN, Murphey-Corb M, Hu FS, Kuebler D, Davison B (1995) Distribution of SIV in lymph nodes of serially sacrificed rhesus monkeys. AIDS Res Hum Retroviruses 11:273
11. Beer B, Scherer J, zur Megede J, Norley S, Baier M, Kurth R (1996) Lack of dichotomy between virus load of peripheral blood and lymph nodes during long-term simian immunodeficiency virus infection of African green monkeys. Virology 219:367
12. Birx DL, Lewis MG, Vahey M, Tencer K, Zack PM, Brown CR, Jahrling PB, Tosato G, Burke D, Redfield R (1993) Association of interleukin-6 in the pathogenesis of acutely fatal SIVsmm/PBj-14 in pigtailed macaques. AIDS Res Hum Retroviruses 9:1123
13. Bonyhadi ML, Rabin L, Salimi S, Brown DA, Kosek J, McCune JM, Kaneshima H (1993) HIV induces thymus depletion in vivo. Nature 363:728
14. Boucher CA, Tersmette M, Lange JM, Kellam P, de Goede RE, Mulder JW, Darby G, Goudsmit J, Larder BA (1990) Zidovudine sensitivity of human immunodeficiency viruses from high-risk, symptom-free individuals during therapy. Lancet 336:585
15. Chakrabarti L, Hurtrel M, Maire MA, Vazeux R, Dormont D, Montagnier L, Hurtrel B (1991) Early viral replication in the brain of SIV-infected rhesus monkeys. Am J Pathol 139:1273
16. Chakrabarti L, Cumont MC, Montagnier L, Hurtrel B (1994) Kinetics of primary SIV infection in lymph nodes. J Med Primatol 23:117
17. Chen ZW, Kou ZC, Shen L, Regan JD, Lord CI, Halloran M, Lee-Parritz D, Fultz PN, Letvin NL (1994) An acutely lethal simian immunodeficiency virus stimulates expansion of V beta 7- and V beta 14-expressing T lymphocytes. Proc Natl Acad Sci USA 91:7501
18. Cocchi F, DeVico AL, Garzino DA, Arya SK, Gallo RC, Lusso P (1995) Identification of RANTES, MIP-1 alpha, and MIP-1 beta as the major HIV-suppressive factors produced by CD8[+] T cells. Science 270:1811
19. Daniel MD, Kirchhoff F, Czajak SC, Sehgal PK, Desrosiers RC (1992) Protective effects of a live attenuated SIV vaccine with a deletion in the nef gene. Science 258:1938
20. Dittmar MT, Cichutek K, Fultz PN, Kurth R (1995) The U3 promoter region of the acutely lethal simian immunodeficiency virus clone smmPBj1.9 confers related biological activity on the apathogenic clone agm3mc. Proc Natl Acad Sci USA 92:1362
21. Dragic T, Litwin V, Allaway GP, Martin SR, Huang YX, Nagashima KA, Cayanan C, Maddon PJ, Koup RA, Moore JP, Paxton WA (1996) HIV-1 entry into CD4(+) cells is mediated by the chemokine receptor CC-CKR-5. Nature 381:667
22. Du Z, Lang SM, Sasseville VG, Lackner AA, Ilyinskii PO, Daniel MD, Jung JU, Desrosiers RC (1995) Identification of a nef allele that causes lymphocyte activation and acute disease in macaque monkeys. Cell 82:665
23. Du Z, Ilyinskii PO, Sasseville VG, Newstein M, Lackner AA, Desrosiers RC (1996) Requirements for lymphocyte activation by unusual strains of simian immunodeficiency virus. J Virol 70:4157
24. Emau P, McClure HM, Isahakia M, Else JG, Fultz PN (1991) Isolation from African Sykes' monkeys (Cercopithecus mitis) of a lentivirus related to human and simian immunodeficiency viruses. J Virol 65:2135
25. Embretson J, Zupancic M, Ribas JL, Burke A, Racz P, Tenner-Racz K, Haase AT (1993) Massive covert infection of helper T lymphocytes and macrophages by HIV during the incubation period of AIDS. Nature 362:359
26. Ennen J, Findeklee H, Dittmar MT, Norley S, Ernst M, Kurth R (1994) CD8[+] T lymphocytes of African green monkeys secrete an immunodeficiency virus-suppressing lymphokine. Proc Natl Acad Sci USA 91:7207
27. Estaquier J, Idziorek T, de Bels F, Barre-Sinoussi F, Hurtrel B, Aubertin AM, Venet A, Mehtali M, Muchmore E, Michel P, Mouton Y, Girard M, Ameisen JC (1994) Programmed cell death and AIDS:

significance of T cell apoptosis in pathogenic and nonpathogenic primate lentiviral infections. Proc Natl Acad Sci USA 91:9431

28. Fauci A (1995) Immunopathogenic mechanisms of human immunodeficiency virus disease: implications for therapy. Am J Med 99 [Suppl 6A]:59

29. Fultz PN (1991) Replication of an acutely lethal simian immunodeficiency virus activates and induces proliferation of lymphocytes. J Virol 65:4902

30. Fultz PN, McClure HM, Anderson DC, Switzer WM (1989) Identification and biologic characterization of an acutely lethal variant of simian immunodeficiency virus from sooty mangabeys (SIV/SMM). AIDS Res Hum Retroviruses 5:397

31. Fultz PN, Stricker RB, McClure HM, Anderson DC, Switzer WM, Horaist C (1990) Humoral response to SIV/SMM infection in macaque and mangabey monkeys. J AIDS 3:319

32. Grant RM, Staprans SI, McClure HM, Johnson RP, Feinberg MB (1995) Viral evolution in sooty mangabeys and rhesus macaques. Abstracts of the 13th Annual Symposium on Nonhuman Primate Models for AIDS, Monterey, CA, USA, November 5–8, 1995. California Regional Primate Research Center, Davis, CA. Abstr. no. 21

33. Groux H, Torpier G, Monte D, Mouton Y, Capron A, Ameisen JC (1992) Activation-induced death by apoptosis in CD4+ T cells from human immunodeficiency virus-infected asymptomatic individuals. J Exp Med 175:331

34. Hartung S, Norley S, Kraus G, Werner A, Vogel M, Bergmann L, Baier M, Kurth R (1990) Infection of non-human primates with SIVagm and HIV-2. In: Schellekens H, Horzinek MC (eds) Animal Models in AIDS. Elsevier, Amsterdam, p 73

35. Hartung S, Boller K, Cichutek K, Norley SG, Kurth R (1992) Quantitation of a lentivirus in its natural host:simian immunodeficiency virus in African green monkeys. J Virol 66:2143

36. Hirsch VM, Olmsted RA, Murphey-Corb M, Purcell RH, Johnson PR (1989) An African primate lentivirus (SIVsm) closely related to HIV-2. Nature 339:389

37. Hirsch VM, Zack PM, Vogel AP, Johnson PR (1991) Simian immunodeficiency virus infection of macaques:end-stage disease is characterized by widespread distribution of proviral DNA in tissues. J Infect Dis 163:976

38. Hirsch VM, Dapolito G, Johnson PR, Elkins WR, London WT, Montali RJ, Goldstein S, Brown C (1995) Induction of AIDS by simian immunodeficiency virus from an African green monkey:species-specific variation in pathogenicity correlates with the extent of in vivo replication. J Virol 69:955

39. Ho DD, Neumann AU, Perelson AS, Chen W, Leonard JM, Markowitz M (1995) Rapid turnover of plasma virions and CD4 lymphocytes in HIV-1 infection. Nature 373:123

40. Hurtrel B, Chakrabarti L, Hurtrel M, Bach JM, Ganiere JP, Montagnier L (1994) Early events in lymph nodes during infection with SIV and FIV. Res Virol 145:221

41. Joag SV, Li Z, Foresman L, Stephens EB, Zhao LJ, Adany I, Pinson DM, McClure HM, Narayan O (1996) Chimeric simian human immunodeficiency virus that causes progressive loss of CD4(+) T cells and AIDS in pig tailed macaques. J Virol 70:3189

42. Kanki PJ, Kurth R, Becker W, Dreesman G, McLane MF, Essex M (1985) Antibodies to simian T lymphotropic retrovirus type III in African green monkeys and recognition of STLV-III viral proteins by AIDS and related sera. Lancet 1:1330

43. Kannagi M, Chalifoux LV, Lord CI, Letvin NL (1988) Suppression of simian immunodeficiency virus replication in vitro by CD8+ lymphocytes. J Immunol 140:2237

44. Kestler HW, Ringler DJ, Mori K, Panicali DL, Sehgal PK, Daniel MD, Desrosiers RC (1991) Importance of the nef gene for maintenance of high virus loads and for development of AIDS. Cell 65:651

45. Lackner AA, Smith MO, Munn RJ, Martfeld DJ, Gardner MB, Marx PA, Dandekar S (1991) Localization of simian immunodeficiency virus in the central nervous system of rhesus monkeys. Am J Pathol 139:609

46. Lackner AA, Vogel P, Ramos RA, Kluge JD, Marthas M (1994) Early events in tissues during infection with pathogenic (SIVmac239) and nonpathogenic (SIVmac1A11) molecular clones of simian immunodeficiency virus. Am J Pathol 145:428

47. Lane TE, Buchmeier MJ, Watry DD, Jakubowski DB, Fox HS (1995) Serial passage of microglial SIV results in selection of homogeneous env quasispecies in the brain. Virology 212:458

48. Lewis MG, Zack PM, Elkins WR, Jahrling PB (1992) Infection of rhesus and cynomolgus macaques with a rapidly fatal SIV (SIVSMM/PBj) isolate from sooty mangabeys. AIDS Res Hum Retroviruses 8:1631

49. Li J, Lord CI, Haseltine W, Letvin NL, Sodroski J (1992) Infection of cynomolgus monkeys with a chimeric HIV-1/SIVmac virus that expresses the HIV-1 envelope glycoproteins. J AIDS 5:639

50. Luciw PA, Prattlowe E, Shaw K, Levy JA, Chengmayer C (1995) Persistent infection of rhesus macaques with T cell-line-tropic and macrophage-tropic clones of simian human immunodeficiency viruses (SHIV). Proc Natl Acad Sci USA 92:7490

51. Mandell CP, Jain NC, Miller CJ, Dandekar S (1995) Bone marrow monocyte/macrophages are an early cellular target of pathogenic and nonpathogenic isolates of Simian immunodeficiency virus (SIVmac) in rhesus macaques. Lab Invest 72:323

52. Manns A, König H, Baier M, Kurth R, Grosse F (1991) Fidelity of reverse transcriptase of the simian immunodeficiency virus from African green monkey. Nucleic Acids Res 19:533

53. Mansfield KG, Pauley D, Young HL, Lackner AA (1995) Mycobacterium avium complex in macaques with AIDS is associated with a specific strain of simian immunodeficiency virus and prolonged survival after primary infection. J Infect Dis 172:1149

54. Marthas ML, van Rompay KK, Otsyula M, Miller CJ, Canfield DR, Pedersen NC, McChesney MB (1995) Viral factors determine progression to AIDS in simian immunodeficiency virus-infected newborn rhesus macaques. J Virol 69:4198

55. Myers G, MacInnes K, Korber B (1992) The emergence of simian/human immunodeficiency viruses. AIDS Res Hum Retroviruses 8:373

56. Norley SG, Kraus G, Ennen J, Bonilla J, Koenig H, Kurth R (1990) Immunological studies of the basis for the apathogenicity of simian immunodeficiency virus from African green monkeys. Proc Natl Acad Sci USA 87:9067

57. Norley S, Beer B, Binninger-Schinzel D, Cosma C, Kurth R (1996) Protection from pathogenic SIVmac challenge following short-term infection with a Nef-deficient attenuated virus. Virology 219:195

58. Novembre FJ, Johnson PR, Lewis MG, Anderson DC, Klumpp S, McClure HM, Hirsch VM (1993) Multiple viral determinants contribute to pathogenicity of the acutely lethal simian immunodeficiency virus SIVsmmPBj variant. J Virol 67:2466

59. Ohta Y, Masuda T, Tsujimoto H, Ishikawa K, Kodama T, Morikawa S, Nakai M, Honjo S, Hayami M (1988) Isolation of simian immunodeficiency virus from African green monkeys and seroepidemiologic survey of the virus in various non-human primates. Int J Cancer 41:115

60. Pantaleo G, Graziosi C, Demarest JF, Butini L, Montroni M, Fox CH, Orenstein JM, Kotler DP, Fauci AS (1993) HIV infection is active and progressive in lymphoid tissue during the clinically latent stage of disease. Nature 362:355

61. Persidsky Y, Steffan AM, Gendrault JL, Hurtrel B, Berger S, Royer C, Stutte HJ, Muchmore E, Aubertin AM, Kirn A (1995) Permissiveness of Kupffer cells for simian immunodeficiency virus (SIV) and morphological changes in the liver of rhesus monkeys at different periods of SIV infection. Hepatology 21:1215

62. Rud EW, Cranage M, Yon J, Quirk J, Ogilvie L, Cook N, Webster S, Dennis M, Clarke BE (1994) Molecular and biological characterization of simian immunodeficiency virus macaque strain 32H proviral clones containing nef size variants. J Gen Virol 75:529

63. Sakuragi S, Shibata R, Mukai R, Komatsu T, Fukasawa M, Sakai H, Sakuragi J, Kawamura M, Ibuki K, Hayami M, Adachi A (1992) Infection of macaque monkeys with a chimeric human and simian immunodeficiency virus. J Gen Virol 7:2983

64. Schmitz J, van LJ, Tenner RK, Grossschupff G, Racz P, Schmitz H, Dietrich M, Hufert FT (1994) Follicular dendritic cells retain HIV-1 particles on their plasma membrane, but are not productively infected in asymptomatic patients with follicular hyperplasia. J Immunol 153:1352

65. Schultz AM, Stott EJ (1994) Primate models for AIDS vaccines. AIDS 8 [Suppl 1]:203

66. Sharer LR, Baskin GB, Cho ES, Murphey-Corb M, Blumberg BM, Epstein LG (1988) Comparison of simian immunodeficiency virus and human immunodeficiency virus encephalitides in the immature host. Ann Neurol 12: S108

67. Simon MA, Brodie SJ, Sasseville VG, Chalifoux LV, Desrosiers RC, Ringler DJ (1994) Immunopathogenesis of SIVmac. Virus Res 32:227

68. Smith MO, Heyes MP, Lackner AA (1995) Early intrathecal events in rhesus macaques (*Macaca mulatta*) infected with pathogenic or nonpathogenic molecular clones of simian immunodeficiency virus. Lab Invest 72:547

69. Villinger F, Lauro S, Folks TM, Ansari AA (1992) Does sequence diversity of the Nef gene contribute to the disease resistance and susceptibility to SIV infection in naturally infected mangabeys and exper-

imentally infected macaques? Abstracts of the 10th Annual Symposium of Nonhum Primate Models for Aids. Puerto Rico, Nov. 17–20, 1992. Puerto Rico Medical School, Puerto Rico. Abstr. no. 17

70. Wei XP, Ghosh SK, Taylor ME, Johnson VA, Emini EA, Deutsch P, Lifson JD, Bonhoeffer S, Nowak MA, Hahn BH, Saag MS, Shaw GM (1995) Viral dynamics in human immunodeficiency virus type 1 infection. Nature 373:117

71. Whatmore AM, Cook N, Hall GA, Sharpe S, Rud EW, Cranage MP (1995) Repair and evolution of nef in vivo modulates simian immunodeficiency virus virulence. J Virol 69:5117

72. Wyand MS, Manson KH, Garciamoll M, Montefiori D, Desrosiers RC (1996) Vaccine protection by a triple deletion mutant of simian immunodeficiency virus. J Virol 70:3724

Springer
and the
environment

At Springer we firmly believe that an international science publisher has a special obligation to the environment, and our corporate policies consistently reflect this conviction.

We also expect our business partners – paper mills, printers, packaging manufacturers, etc. – to commit themselves to using materials and production processes that do not harm the environment. The paper in this book is made from low- or no-chlorine pulp and is acid free, in conformance with international standards for paper permanency.

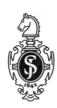 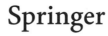

Druck: Strauss Offsetdruck, Mörlenbach
Verarbeitung: Schäffer, Grünstadt